PUTTING
YOUR
PATIENTS
ON THE
PUMP

Karen M. Bolderman
RD, LD, CDE

American Diabetes Association.
Cure • Care • Commitment℠

Director, Book Publishing, John Fedor; *Associate Director, Professional Books,* Christine B. Welch, *Editor;* Joyce Raynor; *Production Manager,* Peggy M. Rote; *Composition,* Circle Graphics, Inc.; *Cover Design,* Koncept, Inc.; *Printer,* Graphic Communications, Inc.

Printed in the United States of America
1 3 5 7 9 10 8 6 4 2

The suggestions and information contained in this publication are generally consistent with the *Clinical Practice Recommendations* and other policies of the American Diabetes Association, but they do not represent the policy or position of the Association or any of its boards or committees. Reasonable steps have been taken to ensure the accuracy of the information presented. However, the American Diabetes Association cannot ensure the safety or efficacy of any product or service described in this publication. Individuals are advised to consult a physician or other appropriate health care professional before undertaking any diet or exercise program or taking any medication referred to in this publication. Professionals must use and apply their own professional judgment, experience, and training and should not rely solely on the information contained in this publication before prescribing any diet, exercise, or medication. The American Diabetes Association—its officers, directors, employees, volunteers, and members—assumes no responsibility or liability for personal or other injury, loss, or damage that may result from the suggestions or information in this publication.

⊗ The paper in this publication meets the requirements of the ANSI Standard Z39.48-1992 (permanence of paper).

ADA titles may be purchased for business or promotional use or for special sales. For information, please write to Lee Romano Sequeira, Special Sales & Promotions, at the address below.

American Diabetes Association
1701 North Beauregard Street
Alexandria, Virginia 22311

Library of Congress Cataloging-in-Publication Data
Bolderman, Karen M., 1954–
    Putting your patients on the pump / Karen M. Bolderman.
        p. cm.
    Includes bibliographical references.
    ISBN 1-58040-148-1 (pbk. : alk. paper)
        1. Insulin pumps. 2. Patient education. 3. Diabetes. I. Title.

RC661.I63 B65 2002
616.4'62061—dc21
                                                                2002066619

To live is the rarest thing in the world; most people exist, that is all.

—OSCAR WILDE

Contents

Foreword

I have been an endocrinologist involved in the management of diabetes for the past 25 years. I began in this task before glucose meters existed. In 1977 when I started the Diabetes Clinic at The Johns Hopkins University School of Medicine, Ames gave me the first Dextrometer to use. It took several minutes to get a reading on a dial the size of a bathroom scale, but what a step forward it was. When insulin pumps became clinically available, I actively championed their use, although the early ones were the size of an Uzi.

I have continued to recommend insulin pumps for my patients over the ensuing years and now have several hundred patients on pumps.

When Karen Bolderman came to work for me many years ago, she was having some difficulty regulating her glucose levels but was not anxious to make the change from multiple daily injections to the pump. One of her most important roles as a diabetes educator in my office was to teach patients how to use their insulin pumps. Together, we developed a system and a philosophy of who should use pump therapy and how a pump should be used. And with time and experience, Karen finally decided that the pump would be good for her. Based on the book that follows, you will see that she is sold on the value of insulin pump therapy.

Not surprisingly, Karen and I have very similar ideas on who are pump candidates, how to start patients on pumps, and how to adjust basal and bolus insulin doses for optimal control. In the subsequent pages, you will learn what we have come to learn over many years of trial and error, through review of the literature and extensive personal experience. Karen is one of the best diabetes educators I have ever worked with. The lessons to be learned in *Putting Your Patients on the Pump* will help any health care provider to make the most of insulin pump therapy, all with the goal of improving the life of the person with diabetes.

Read ahead and enjoy.

James H. Mersey, MD
Director, Endocrinology and Metabolism,
Greater Baltimore Medical Center
Assistant Professor of Medicine,
The Johns Hopkins University School of Medicine
Clinical Associate Professor of Medicine,
University of Maryland School of Medicine,
Baltimore, Maryland

Preface

Insulin pump therapy gives people with diabetes the freedom to enjoy life, despite their chronic condition. The value and importance of having freedom is obvious from the impact this innovative technology has made in just 25 years: The insulin pump is now a common, integral component of diabetes management.

As a long-term insulin pump wearer and a health care professional who has learned much from my colleagues and countless other "pumpers," I have a unique perspective and understand what constitutes practical, useful information. This book will help health care professionals with expertise in diabetes care successfully start and maintain diabetes patients on insulin pump therapy. I believe that even experienced clinicians will find the checklists for patients and the ideas on staging the patient selection and education processes helpful.

I hope this book supports the extra efforts diabetes health care professionals must make to help their patients achieve success using an insulin pump.

Acknowledgments

I wanted to be a teacher for as long as I can remember. When I developed diabetes in 1965, my parents, physicians, and teachers encouraged me to learn all that I could about diabetes and to fit diabetes into my life—not build my life around diabetes. Years later, insulin pump therapy made my life with diabetes much easier, and I wanted others to benefit from my experience.

Many people have had an impact on my career as a diabetes educator as well as my life with diabetes. I owe much to my personal physician, G. William Benedict, MD, for his guidance and patience in putting *me* on my first pump many years ago. I am also beholden to Jim Mersey, MD, Chief of Endocrinology at Greater Baltimore Medical Center (GBMC) and Medical Director of the Geckle Diabetes and Nutrition Center at GBMC, Baltimore, Maryland, for providing me with unique and rewarding career opportunities and for teaching me the finer points of diabetes management. I am honored that he agreed to write the Foreword to this book.

A special thank you goes out to the reviewers Bonnie Brost, RD, LD, CDE; Nathaniel Clark, MS, RD, MD; Charlene Freeman, RN, CDE; and David Schade, MD, for kindly providing their time and expertise.

I want to thank the American Diabetes Association for providing me with the opportunity to write this book. I am especially indebted to Christine Welch, Associate Director, Professional Books,

American Diabetes Association, and book editors Joyce Raynor and Wendy Martin for their dedicated editorial work, insight, and ongoing support.

A note of acknowledgment is also extended to my colleagues Linda Egeto, RN, and Lynn Senecal, RD, CDE, for sharing their experience and wisdom. In addition, I thank Hope Warshaw, MMSc, RD, CDE, for her friendship and literary guidance. I extend gratitude also to my loving and very patient husband and family for their constant support and encouragement and to my professional colleagues through my years as a pump therapy diabetes educator. I am especially thankful to Frank Weller (d, 1997); Scott Fischell; Cindy Shump, RN, MS, MSN, CRNP, CDE; Zoe Myers, MA; James Dicke, MD; and Joanna Tyzack, MD.

Thanks also go out to the countless pump patients with whom I have had the pleasure to work and learn from. Their contribution to my knowledge of diabetes has been of untold value, for which I am most grateful.

CHAPTER 1

Insulin Pump Therapy Benefits and Challenges

Insulin pump therapy is in its third decade and is gaining wider popularity. There are more than 120,000 diabetes patients now using an insulin pump. Until research yields a practical way to replace lost β-cell function in diabetes, the insulin pump provides the most elegant method of insulin replacement. In its best application, pump therapy is a rare win-win situation in diabetes in terms of glycemic control and personal freedom.

An insulin pump is a wonderful diabetes management tool, but as with any tool, the pump is only as good as the patient's ability to use it. Clinicians have a responsibility to carefully screen and teach all patients who express an interest in pump therapy. When patients are mismatched with the pump, or the pump regimen, potential benefits are lost or nullified.

Insulin pump: A small, programmable, and external battery-powered device that delivers insulin in tiny continuous amounts (basal doses) and in larger amounts for meals (bolus doses). The pump is attached to the patient by an infusion set consisting of long, thin flexible tubing with a needle or catheter on the end that is inserted subcutaneously into the patient. The user programs and operates the pump to deliver insulin doses that match individual needs.

Successful pump therapy is more likely with motivated and conscientious patients. Regardless of what many patients first think, the pump patient must perform frequent self-monitoring of blood glucose (SMBG) to ensure proper pump function and document glucose control. Also, the patient must calculate insulin-to-carbohydrate ratios to determine how much food-related bolus insulin he or she requires.

MYTHS OF INSULIN PUMP THERAPY

Patient	Provider
No more SMBG	Any patient can use a pump
Can eat whenever I want	Less emphasis on meal planning
Can eat as much as I want	Not useful in type 2 diabetes
Too expensive	Too expensive
Too much trouble	Too complicated for most

The education in pump use provided by the health care professional is crucial in correcting any misconceptions the patient may have about pump therapy and, even more important, in guiding the patient as he or she develops pump skills. The truth about pump therapy is that the greater the patient's effort, the greater the chance that therapy will succeed.

BENEFITS

For People with Type 1 Diabetes

- Improves glycemic control by delivering an individualized basal rate supplemented with bolus doses to match the patient's intake and correct any hyperglycemia. Erratic glucose fluctuations are greatly reduced
- Offers precise dosage delivery in basal rates as low as 0.05 units/h and bolus doses in exact whole and tenth-unit doses
- Can be programmed to manage the dawn phenomenon by delivering a higher basal rate during the dawn hours[1]
- Can be programmed to control glucose during and after exercise by delivering a lower basal rate
- Decreases the risk of hypoglycemia by allowing patients to individualize insulin doses to match their requirements hour by hour

- May lessen or reverse hypoglycemia unawareness by decreasing the incidence of hypoglycemia
- Allows incremental, precise doses to match growth spurts in children and adolescents[2] and to manage people who are insulin sensitive
- Improves gastroparesis management with the option of splitting and/or extending bolus delivery over time to match delayed absorption of nutrients
- Eliminates the frequency and inconvenience of multiple daily injections
- Increases lifestyle flexibility by allowing the person to eat at desired intervals of time instead of matching food intake to injection therapy insulin peak times
- Improves well-being and quality of life by providing freedom in school, work, exercise, and leisure-time schedule variations
- Allows for easier weight loss. With individualized dosing, the pump patient is not "chasing insulin" with additional food.

For People with Type 2 Diabetes

- Allows the attainment and maintenance of improved glycemic control
- Eliminates the frequency and inconvenience of multiple daily injections
- Increases lifestyle flexibility by allowing the person to eat at desired intervals of time instead of matching food intake to injection therapy insulin peak times[3]
- Improves well-being and quality of life by providing freedom in school, work, exercise, and leisure-time schedule variations
- Allows for easier weight loss. With individualized dosing, the pump patient is not "chasing insulin" with additional food.

For Women Who Are Pregnant or Planning Pregnancy

- Mimics normal physiology with individualized precise dosage delivery
- Decreases pre- and postprandial glucose (PPG) excursions
- Reduces risk of hypoglycemia
- Improves the management of morning sickness by eliminating the need to eat on rising: a correctly calculated basal rate maintains euglycemia
- Allows for easier achievement of recommended tight blood glucose goals.

▨ Reduces postprandial hyperglycemia due to the delayed gastric emptying of normal pregnancy as well as gastropathy with the use of the extended, square-wave, or combination bolus feature.[4]

THE DOWNSIDE

Pump therapy is not without some drawbacks, although a patient with motivation and training can tackle practically any drawback. However, inattention to problems can create life-threatening circumstances. Weigh these drawbacks against the benefits.

▨ **A learning curve.** Pump therapy requires education, skills training, and initial intensive follow-up and management. **A patient contemplating pump therapy must know beforehand how to count carbohydrate and match insulin doses with carbohydrate intake and basal needs.** The pump wearer must learn the technical "buttonology" of their specific pump and learn how to fill the insulin cartridge/reservoir, change the tubing and infusion set, and calculate appropriate insulin bolus doses. Intensive follow-up for the first few weeks after pump initiation is essential and includes detailed record keeping of glucose levels, carbohydrate intake, exercise, and insulin doses. For children, the learning curve also involves their parents and caregivers.

▨ **Frequent SMBG.** The pump wearer must perform a minimum of four glucose checks daily, with additional checks as needed between meals; during sleep hours; before, during, and after exercise; during illness and at times of stress; and when glucose levels become erratic. Bolus doses of insulin must be calculated to match the person's food intake, anticipated activity, and current glucose level.

▨ **Possible weight gain.** Insulin pumps offer precise dosage delivery to match the patient's food intake. It can become easy for the pump wearer to bolus extra insulin for additional calories. People may begin to eat foods that may have been considered "forbidden" before using a pump and may overindulge in high-calorie foods of low nutrient value. Although glycemic control can be maintained with additional insulin doses for excessive caloric intake, weight gain can result.

■ **Hypoglycemia.** If the basal rates are not set correctly or if the pump wearer miscalculates and overdoses a bolus delivery or doesn't compensate for exercise, hypoglycemia can result. Pattern management is very important.

■ **Unexpected hyperglycemia.** If the patient miscalculates or improperly sets the basal rate(s) or bolus doses, hyperglycemia can go uncorrected. The rare pump failure or occasional site occlusion can decrease or prevent basal/bolus delivery, resulting in hyperglycemia.

■ **Ketoacidosis.** In addition to the potential improper setting of the basal rate(s), pump malfunction may also cause partial or total interruption in the basal delivery. Because the pump uses only rapid- or short-acting (regular) insulin, there is no "background" insulin available for hyperglycemia and the prevention of ketones. Studies from the early 1980s and 1990s revealed a decrease in diabetic ketoacidosis in pump wearers.[5,6]

■ **Skin irritation and infusion site infections.** People with sensitive skin may develop redness, tenderness, itching, or rashes from the infusion set tape. Those who perspire heavily or participate in water sports may have problems with getting the tape to stick to their skin. Removing the adhesive may also cause concern. Site infections can occur from poor insertion technique or leaving the infusion set in place too long.

■ **Logistics/placement.** Although the insulin pump weighs about 4 oz and is the size of a beeper, wearing it creates challenges. Despite offering flexibility in lifestyle, many people may find it unpleasant or intolerable to be connected 24 h a day to a small external device. Pumps require a clip, a case with a built-in clip, or a belt-loop case for attachment. Some people prefer to place their pump in a pocket, whereas others may choose to wear their pump discreetly under clothing. Intimacy, showering or bathing, exercise, and contact sports create additional challenges in how to wear the pump.

■ **Paying for it.** In 2002, the average price of an insulin pump is between $5,000 and $6,000. Disposable supplies, including pump batteries, insulin cartridges/reservoirs, infusion sets, and skin preparation products can add up to an additional $1,500 or more per year. Some insurance companies cover all or some of the expense, whereas others may provide for only the pump and not the supplies, or vice versa.

CHAPTER 2

Candidate Selection

Many patients are naturals for pump therapy, but it is not for everyone. Some need to overcome specific obstacles before the pump will be an asset to their health care. Others just do not have the interest or abilities to master pump therapy. Discovering the character and source of motivation through careful screening of the patient is the key to ensuring success in pump therapy.

You must evaluate the physical and psychological readiness of each pump candidate to take on the responsibilities and challenges of pump therapy. The person with diabetes and his or her family need to buy into pump therapy. Input from the patient's family and other members of the health care team will help you discern the patient's clinical and lifestyle indications for insulin pump therapy (Table 1).

PROFILE OF A GOOD PROSPECT: READY, WILLING, AND ABLE

- **Is motivated.** Pump therapy requires readiness, preparedness, and a time investment for weeks or months in advance and during the initiation of pump therapy.

- **Has realistic expectations.** The patient who expresses interest and desire for pump therapy must understand that the pump

TABLE 1.   Indications for Pump Therapy

Clinical indications	Lifestyle indications
▪ Inadequate glycemic control with MDI therapy	▪ Erratic schedule
▪ Recurrent hypoglycemia	▪ Varied work shifts
▪ Recurrent hyperglycemia	▪ Desire for flexibility
▪ Hypoglycemia unawareness	▪ Inconvenience of multiple-dose
▪ Dawn phenomenon	injections
▪ Preconception	
▪ Pregnancy	
▪ Gastroparesis	
▪ Early neuropathy or nephropathy, when improvement in glucose control can reduce acceleration of complications	
▪ Renal transplantation	

will not "fix" blood glucose variations automatically, nor will pump therapy grant freedom from frequent SMBG. Pump therapy does not guarantee "good control," but it can help achieve and maintain good glucose control with effort from the pump wearer. Children who use the pump must have parents and caretakers with a thorough understanding of what pump therapy involves and the willingness to spend the time needed working with the child and health care professionals.

■ **Demonstrates independent diabetes management.** Ideally, multiple daily injection (MDI) therapy precedes pump therapy. MDI as a "stepping stone" to pump therapy often reveals the patient's suitability. At the very minimum, the prospective pump user should have knowledge of the basics of diabetes education, including all topics listed in the National Standards for Diabetes Self-Management Education.[7] A thorough knowledge of diabetes and its management and the ability to demonstrate appropriate self-care behaviors provide the foundation for the advanced self-management skills required by pump users. This is one of the reasons pump therapy is not recommended for newly diagnosed patients.[8]

■ **Is willing to learn.** The person must be able and willing to learn, practice, and demonstrate an understanding of carbohydrate counting, insulin action, and premeal bolus dose calculations and be able to make insulin dose adjustments in response to hypoglycemia and hyperglycemia.

■ **Welcomes challenges.** The initial few weeks of pump therapy require detailed record keeping of SMBG results, dietary intake, insulin doses, and exercise, as well as frequent (minimum of four daily) blood glucose checks, including "middle of the night" checks (typically at 3:00 a.m.), and daily telephone/fax communication with the health care professional(s). The pump user must also be comfortable with using needles and have patience during the pump initiation period, when appropriate basal rates and insulin-to-carbohydrate ratios are being determined.

■ **Has the support of family or significant other.** The decision to initiate pump therapy is a lifestyle-changing decision. Emotional support is crucial to the success of pump therapy. Family members, friends, coworkers, teachers, and others can be of great assistance to the pump wearer. Education about diabetes in general, along with pump therapy education can help ease the difficulties and challenges of the pump therapy initiation.

■ **Can afford it.** Pumps and pump supplies cost thousands of dollars, so verifying the patient's ability to afford pump therapy is essential. The pump wearer must have either personal resources or adequate insurance benefits. Insurance coverage can range from 50 to 100% for the pump and/or pump supplies. Ask the potential pump wearer to verify their benefits with their health insurance carrier; some pump manufacturers will provide this service to patients. Some insurance companies cover only a specific brand of pump but may provide benefits for a nonformulary brand with a letter of medical necessity from the prescribing physician. Medicare covers pumps for patients with both type 1 and type 2 diabetes who perform at least 4 SMBG checks and use at least 3 injections per day but requires documentation including specific C-peptide criteria. At present, the C-peptide must be ≤110% of the low range (e.g., up to and including 0.99 ng/ml, if the low range is 0.9 ng/ml).

■ **Is capable intellectually, physically, and technically.** A patient contemplating pump therapy must be able to demonstrate an understanding of the therapy. The ability to wear the pump, fill and/or place the insulin cartridge/reservoir into the pump, and perform the technical functions of the pump is essential.

- Patients with moderate to severe hand arthritis or neuropathy may not be able to press the pump's buttons or handle the insulin cartridge/reservoir and infusion sets.
- Patients who are blind or visually impaired may be limited in their choice of pump because of a lack of audio functions.
- Patients with hearing loss may be at greater risk for interruptions in insulin delivery because they have difficulty hearing the pump's alarm. Patients who are deaf can use pumps with vibrating alarms.

Demonstrates emotional stability. The pump patient must routinely attend education sessions and attend to tasks that require routine. A patient with untreated depression, eating disorders, manipulative behavior, or other psychoses is usually ill-suited for pump therapy. Carefully assess the pump candidate's psychological status, or refer the patient to a mental health professional. Suggest treatment options for behaviors that may interfere with pump therapy.

CONTRAINDICATIONS

Although pump therapy does not increase the risk of mortality among its users,[8] the frequency of adverse events increases with:

- Poor candidate selection
- Insufficient or inadequate supervision and monitoring by the diabetes health care professional or team
- Infrequent SMBG
- Inexperienced practitioners

Young or old, age in itself is not necessarily a contraindication to successful pump therapy. Children as young as newborns and people in their 70s have achieved success with pump therapy.

STEPS FOR HELPING THE PATIENT DECIDE

You may be able to identify good candidates for insulin pump therapy, but patients still need to decide whether pump therapy is for them. Here is an education plan for helping the patient make this decision.

1. Give the patient a general overview of what pump therapy entails. Discuss the advantages and challenges, as well as realistic goals and expectations for pump therapy.

2. Review the prospective pump user's medical history and evaluate his or her diabetes knowledge. Consider using written pre- and posttests.

3. Demonstrate how an insulin pump works (bolus delivery). Explain basic pump therapy terms, including basal rate, bolus dose, infusion set, infusion sites, dressing, and insulin cartridge/reservoir. Show available models, and encourage the patient to learn the features offered by each brand of pump. Explain that he or she can disconnect the pump for bathing, intimacy, and intensive sports.

4. Have the patient handle a pump. Some patients mistakenly believe the pump is worn only during the day and removed at bedtime. Others believe an insulin pump is surgically implanted or permanently attached. Most people are surprised to learn how small a pump is and how it is worn.

5. Demonstrate the available infusion sets, e.g., needle versus Teflon cannula and disconnect versus nondisconnect. Explain that tubing is available in various lengths to accommodate where the pump is worn. Show how the pump is worn under clothing, such as in a sock, bra, or pantyhose. Show pump accessories, such as clips, leather cases, fanny bag–type cases, clothing with built-in pump pouches or pockets, and Velcro-attached removable pockets or socks.

6. Demonstrate the insertion and removal of an infusion set. Allow the patient to practice a self-insertion. There is a commercially available injection pad, or "rubber belly," that attaches to the patient's abdomen, thigh, or upper arm with an adjustable strap. Does the patient want to wear an infusion set for a few days to get accustomed to the feel of it? Offer the option of wearing the pump with saline for a few days to determine how the patient likes that pump in particular and pump therapy in general (see Chapter 4). When parents are considering pump therapy for their child, this experience sometimes results in postponing pump therapy; the parents recognize the learning curve and time commitment a pump requires, or they discover that their child is not quite ready. Because saline is a prescription item, the prescribing physician will need to provide a "saline-start" order and a prescription for saline. Pump manufacturer personnel—either a Certified Pump Trainer or clinical staff—will provide brief training on the pump. (For a discussion of how saline can be used during the pump therapy education process, see

Chapter 4.) Some patients see or wear two or three brands of pumps before making a final decision.

7. Provide a list of the various pump manufacturers with names and telephone numbers of the local sales representative, corporate office telephone numbers, and website information. Encourage the patient to contact the manufacturers' sales representatives, who will offer "sales calls" to patients and/or provide literature and a video. Does your protocol place the responsibility of contacting pump manufacturer sales representatives on you? Is there a local pump support group meeting that the patient can attend to meet pump users?

CHAPTER 3

Pump
Selection

Several manufacturers sell insulin pumps, and some offer more than one model. Each pump has slightly different features.

Experience with one brand of pump may bias a physician or educator toward that pump even when another brand or model may suit the patient as well, or better. Sometimes clinicians assume that their personal preferences for pump features are the same as the patient's. As much as possible, allow the patient to choose a pump.

Deciding on a suitable choice usually takes time. Give the patient enough time to view the various pump manufacturer videos, read the marketing literature, review diabetes publications comparison lists and articles about pumps, and meet with the pump manufacturer sales representatives and clinical staff.

PUMP CRITERIA CHECKLIST

General

- Ease of navigating on-screen selections
- Use of icons, words, or abbreviations
- How much memorization is required? Is it difficult to remember how to move from one screen or function to another?
- For a child, could someone only slightly familiar with the pump stop it or perform troubleshooting?

- Ease of manual tasks: Could a user with hand arthritis, carpal tunnel syndrome, or neuropathy use the pump easily?
- How many steps are involved in changing or entering a program?
- Are batteries easy to obtain and replace?
- What type of clock is available, 12-h or 24-h?
- Does the pump have multi-language capacity?
- What is involved in detaching the pump?
- Does the pump have a backlight?
- Is the pump waterproof or watertight? Does it require any special accessories to make it waterproof?
- What is the size of the pump? How thin is the pump? Can it be worn discreetly under clothing?
- How much does the pump weigh?
- How is the pump attached to the person? Are there options, including a removable clip, a case with a built-in clip, a case with built-in belt loops, or a choice of other cases? Is the case available in a variety of colors and materials (leather, vinyl, plastic, etc.)?
- Is the pump available in more than one color? If not, can the user change the outside color or appearance of the pump?

Insulin delivery

- Some pumps make noise during basal and bolus deliveries. Does this matter to the user? Pumps with a solenoid motor make a clicking noise, and those with a direct current motor are virtually noiseless.
- Frequent insulin delivery is an important issue for infants, toddlers, children, and insulin-sensitive adults. If the infusion set cannula or needle is not infusing insulin constantly, subcutaneous or scar tissue may build up and occlude the site, impeding basal delivery. In contrast to pumps with solenoid motors, a direct current motor pump delivers fractions of any basal rate, no matter how high or low, in "micro" pulses every 3 min. Insulin-sensitive patients are better matched to direct current motor pumps.
- Does the basal rate deliver in increments of 0.10 (tenth of a unit) or 0.05 (twentieth of a unit)? Smaller increments are useful for fine-tuning basal rate delivery in children and insulin-sensitive people.

■ Can the user temporarily increase and decrease basal rate delivery, and for how long? Can the pump be programmed to automatically calculate increases or decreases in percentages for several different basal rates, or must the user calculate the basal rate changes manually and then program the pump with the calculated changes? A temporary basal increase is helpful for acute illness or preceding menstruation, whereas a temporary decrease in basal delivery is useful for exercise.

■ How many 24-h basal rate programs can the pump hold? This is useful for patients who want to accommodate activity levels that vary day-to-day. For example, if weekend activity levels are different from weekday activity levels, the user may want to pre-set different 24-h basal programs with higher or lower rates instead of frequently resetting temporary basal rates. The ability to set alternate 24-h basal programs is a helpful feature for children who have gym class on specific days, adults who exercise on alternate days, and patients who are shift workers or weekend athletes, and is also useful for times of premenstrual syndrome, stress, and illness.

■ What types of bolus delivery options does the pump have? Is the bolus delivery increment in tenths, halves, or whole-unit increments, or does the user have a choice? Patients who are insulin sensitive may prefer or require tenth-unit bolus increments.

■ Is there an audio or remote option for patients who want to wear the pump discreetly?

■ Is there more than one type of bolus delivery available? A delayed bolus delivery is useful for gastroparesis and also may be used for high-protein, high-fat meals. How long can delivery be delayed?

■ Does the pump store a history of bolus deliveries? How many? Can this information be downloaded to track trends and patterns of use and dosages?

Safety

■ Can a bolus dose be stopped easily mid-delivery? Can the user track exactly how much bolus was delivered before it was halted?

■ Is there a maximum use lockout feature for children, so that a basal rate or bolus delivery cannot be programmed for more than a specific upper limit?

- Is there a time-out feature that the user can pre-set to halt all insulin delivery if a button is not pushed for a specific duration of time?
- What type of safety and performance checks does the pump have? How often does the pump perform self-checks?
- What types of warning and alarm systems does the pump have? Is there an alarm for undelivered basal insulin?
- Does the pump alarm sound when insulin is running low or the cartridge/reservoir is empty? How is the amount indicated? Is it approximate or exact?
- If batteries are removed for an extended period of time, does the pump retain its memory of programmed basal rates and history of bolus doses and alarms?
- Is the warning and/or alarm signal visual, auditory, or tactile? If audio, how loud is it? Patients may need a pump with vibrating warnings and alarms.
- In case of a major technical problem, is a backup pump provided? What are the procedures to obtain a backup pump if one is not provided at the time of purchase? How quickly does the patient receive the replacement pump?
- What is the repair policy? If the pump is returned for problems, is it repaired and reissued to the patient, or is a new pump provided? Are refurbished pumps redistributed?

CUSTOMER SERVICE AND OTHER PRACTICAL CONSIDERATIONS

The pump manufacturer sales personnel should explain the start-to-finish process to both the potential pump user and to his or her health care professional or team. The pump patient must be confident that technical support and assistance is available 24 h a day, 7 days a week. All pumps should have the company's toll-free customer service number displayed on the back.

Another consideration is the procedure for ordering supplies. The pump wearer should know what types of infusion sets, accessories, batteries, and specific pump items, such as cartridges/syringes, are needed. Are replacement supplies obtained, locally or by mail from the pump manufacturer? Some manufacturers offer to send the patient supplies routinely and automatically. What role does the manufacturer play in obtaining insurance coverage for supplies?

On average, an insulin pump costs between $5,000 and $6,000, and most come with a 4-year warranty. Supplies, including batteries, pump cartridges/syringes, infusion sets, skin prep items, and tape, can cost in excess of $1,500 each year. Help the patient understand the price of both the pump and supplies. Insurance coverage ranges from 50 to 100%, with most averaging about 80% coverage. Some insurance companies may provide coverage for the pump but not the supplies, or vice versa.

The pump manufacturer should give a detailed cost estimate in writing to the patient. Usually, a pump manufacturer insurance specialist handles this process. Next, the patient is required to sign an assignment of benefits document, allowing the pump manufacturer to determine the type and amount of insurance coverage provided. This can take 1 day to several weeks to process. An insulin pump is a prescription item, and the prescribing physician must provide the prescription and/or an order for an insulin pump to the patient and/or insurance company. Some insurance companies require a letter of medical necessity from the prescribing physician with additional documentation, which may include:

- Several weeks or months of SMBG records
- Recent glycated hemoglobin A1C (A1C) levels
- Reasons why an insulin pump may be necessary, e.g., erratic glucose pattern correction, preconception, pregnancy, diabetes complications requiring improvement in control, or lifestyle change

It is not uncommon for insurance companies to have a contract with a specified pump manufacturer. Patients who decide on an alternative brand usually need a letter or certificate of medical necessity from the prescribing physician explaining why another pump brand is preferred or required. Because this delays purchase and shipment of the pump, many clinicians have developed form letters to expedite the insurance approval and appeal process. Even if not initially covered, persistence can lead to a noncontract or nonformulary pump approval. Some patients pursue insulin pump insurance coverage for several brands of pumps and opt to settle for the pump that costs the least amount of money. Other patients are firm in their choice and are willing to provide whatever documentation the insurance company may require to approve a noncontract or nonformulary pump.

Patients can request that the company ship the insulin pump directly to the home. However, overzealous and excited patients have been known to self-initiate pump therapy without formal training and have ended up in the emergency room in DKA or hypoglycemic shock. For this reason, some clinicians and diabetes educators request that the company ship a new pump to their site rather than to the patient's home and insist that pump manufacturers provide scheduled formal pump training.

CHAPTER 4

Prepping Pump Patients

Formal training of the patient to use a pump has three stages: pre-pump education, pump start-up, and follow-up and management. Prepump education is usually spread over a few weeks, with a minimum of three visits of 1–3 h each. The usual pump start-up (see Chapter 5) consists of one 3- to 4-h session. Pump follow-up and management can range from a few weeks to several months.

When planning the prepump education, consider the learning style of each individual. Some pump patients complete just three 1-h preparation sessions with a verbal exchange of information, whereas others need a structured learning situation, such as several 1- to 3-h classes spread over 3–4 months, with written tests to gauge the information flow. The average patient will find the latter a bit much. A combination of individual and group sessions may work well because many patients benefit from group interaction. Success begets success, and clinicians are likely to design and implement what they have found works best for their patients.

A group class covering some of the pump education topics can also be time-efficient for the health care professional or team. Ideally, patients should have sessions with an endocrinologist, a diabetes educator (an RN or RD or RPh, Certified Diabetes Educator [CDE]), a dietitian (RD, preferably CDE), and a mental health professional, preferably one with expertise in diabetes.

There are particular education components that will guarantee successful pump therapy. Although the patient's education begins as you present the "Steps for Helping the Patient Decide" (Chapter 2), once a decision to proceed with pump therapy occurs, new educational objectives emerge:

- Establishing goals
- Learning carbohydrate counting
- Calculating insulin-to-carbohydrate ratios
- Managing hyperglycemia and hypoglycemia
- Choosing and inserting infusion sets
- Coping with lifestyle issues, sick days, exercise, supplies, and travel

A patient reference published by the American Diabetes Association, *Putting Your Diabetes on the Pump*,[9] can be of great assistance to your patients as they learn the details of pump therapy.

GOALS

Review or establish appropriate blood glucose and A1C targets with the patient at this time (Table 2).[10] Emphasize that pump therapy does not guarantee an automatic improvement in control but may make achieving control easier while providing a more flexible lifestyle. The responsibility for the improvements patients make using this new tool rests in their hands. Patients who are not doing well on MDI therapy may embrace the greater lifestyle flexibility offered by insulin pump therapy and become willing to put forth the effort needed for success.

Discuss how critical it is for the patient to keep detailed records during the prepump education and pump start-up periods, which could last 1–4 months or longer. SMBG should include frequent pre- and postprandial blood glucose checks, at least four times a day, including one middle-of-the-night check around 3:00 a.m.

For enhanced pattern recognition purposes, ask the patient to also record factors that affect blood glucose, such as:

- Dietary intake, including grams of carbohydrate at each meal and snack
- Insulin doses (basal rates and bolus doses)
- Exercise: intensity, duration, and time of day
- Stress
- Illness
- Menstrual cycle

TABLE 2. Glycemic Control for People with Diabetes*

	Normal	Goal	Additional action suggested
Plasma values			
Average preprandial glucose (mg/dl)	<110	90–130	<90 or >150
Average bedtime glucose (mg/dl)	<120	110–150	<110 or >180
2 h after start of meals (mg/dl)		170–190[†]	
Whole-blood values			
Average preprandial glucose (mg/dl)	<100	80–120	<80 or >140
Average bedtime glucose (mg/dl)	<110	100–140	<100 or >160
2 h after start of meals (mg/dl)		160–180[†]	
A1C (%)	<6	<7	>8

*These values are by necessity generalized to the entire population of individuals with diabetes and are for nonpregnant adults. Patients with comorbid disease, the very young and older adults, and others with unusual conditions or circumstances may warrant different treatment goals. Values above/below these levels are not "goals" nor are they "acceptable" in most patients. They are an indication for a significant change in the treatment plan. "Additional action suggested" depends on individual patient circumstances. Such actions may include enhanced diabetes self-management education, comanagement with a diabetes team, referral to an endocrinologist, change in pharmacological therapy, initiation of or increase in SMBG, or more frequent contact with the patient. A1C is referenced to a nondiabetic range of 4–6%.

†These recommendations come from consensus among diabetes care providers. No American Diabetes Association recommendation exists for postprandial glucose levels.[6]

Remind the patient of the learning curve associated with something as new and detailed as pump therapy initiation. Make assurances that, with time and experience, the patient will earn the freedom of being able to interpret his or her results and make safe self-management decisions.

CARBOHYDRATE COUNTING

It is essential that the patient, or parents if the patient is a child, master carbohydrate counting before beginning pump therapy. This requires instruction from an RD, preferably a CDE with pump therapy experience, and usually takes a few weeks to teach, depending on the patient's history and abilities. Use follow-up session(s) to validate the patient's ability to count carbohydrates accurately. For additional information, refer to the American Diabetes Association book *Practical Carbohydrate Counting: A How-to-Teach Guide for Health Professionals.*[11]

Calculating insulin-to-carbohydrate ratios

A patient's insulin-to-carbohydrate ratio reflects his or her sensitivity to insulin. Generally, the more sensitive a person is to insulin, the higher the insulin-to-carbohydrate ratio. A patient in whom 1 unit of insulin covers 20 g carbohydrate is more insulin sensitive than a patient in whom 1 unit of insulin covers 12 g carbohydrate. Also, because some people are more or less insulin resistant at different times of day or have different levels of activity during the day, they may need to work with more than one ratio.

Insulin-to-carbohydrate ratios are best determined by the RD/CDE during the carbohydrate counting teaching process or can be provided to the patient as a starting point by the prescribing physician or CDE. Pump manufacturers may also provide a CDE to determine insulin-to-carbohydrate ratio and insulin sensitivity factor calculations.

The ratios can be calculated with one of the methods described below. Use whichever method seems most appropriate based on the information you have available. It is a good idea to use one method to determine the insulin-to-carbohydrate ratio and another method to validate the ratio.

Method 1: Food diary, insulin dose, and SMBG information
This method is based on the amount of insulin used to cover consumed carbohydrate. Ask the patient to keep 3–7 days of records, including:

1. Fasting, premeal, and 2-h PPG results
2. Premeal insulin doses
3. Amount of carbohydrate consumed at meals and other times. It is helpful if the patient consumes the same amount of carbohydrate at each breakfast for the week, same amount of carbohydrate at each lunch for the week, etc., until the meal ratio is established.
4. Amount of all food and beverage consumed, because fat, alcohol, and excessive protein (>4 oz) may affect PPG levels.

With these records, determine the amount of insulin the patient used to cover the carbohydrate consumed at each meal by dividing the total grams of carbohydrate by the number of units of insulin.[11]

Example
- Consumed 60 g carbohydrate
- Used 5 units rapid- or short-acting insulin
- PPG was within target range
- $60 \div 5 = 12$
- Insulin-to-carbohydrate ratio = 1:12
- 1 unit of insulin covers 12 g carbohydrate

This method is most effective if SMBG records indicate that the patient is usually within his or her PPG targets. If blood glucose is generally not in control and carbohydrate intake is varied, this method will be less useful because frequent adjustments will be needed.

Method 2: The rule of 500

This rule of thumb, widely used by clinicians to determine the insulin-to-carbohydrate ratio,[6] is based on total (i.e., basal and bolus) daily insulin dose (TDD). The TDD is divided into 500 and the result is the amount of carbohydrate that one unit of rapid- or short-acting insulin will cover, bringing blood glucose into the target range about 3–4 h after the meal.

Example
- TDD is 36 units
- Glucose levels are within target range
- 500 ÷ 36 = 13.8 (round up to 14 or 15)
- Insulin-to-carbohydrate ratio is 1:15
- 1 unit of insulin covers 15 g carbohydrate

Some clinicians find that dividing 450 (rather than 500) by the TDD is more accurate for short-acting insulin and/or for people who are more insulin resistant (i.e., need more insulin to cover carbohydrate).

Method 3: Using the insulin sensitivity factor

The insulin sensitivity factor (ISF) is the amount of blood glucose (in mg/dl) reduced by 1 unit of rapid- or short-acting insulin over 2–4 h.[12] Two commonly accepted formulas are used to determine the ISF: the 1800 Rule and the 1500 Rule. They apply a mathematical constant that expresses the relationship between body size and insulin action. Endocrinologist Paul C. Davidson, MD, from Atlanta, Georgia, developed the 1500 Rule. With the introduction of rapid-acting insulin, John Walsh, PA, CDE, a pump specialist from Escondido, California, modified the 1500 Rule into the 1800 Rule.[6] Clinicians tend to use the 1800 Rule for patients who are insulin sensitive or use rapid-acting insulin and the 1500 Rule for patients who are insulin resistant or use short-acting insulin. Again, trial and error will determine which formula works best in your practice.

The rules calculate the ISF by dividing either 1800 or 1500 by the TDD.

Example 1
- TDD is 34 units

■ $1800 \div 34 = 52.9$

■ ISF is 52.9 mg/dl. One unit of rapid-acting insulin decreases glucose by 52.9 mg/dl. You may round up to 53, but it may be easier to round up to 55 or 60.

Example 2

■ TDD is 34 units

■ $1500 \div 34 = 44$

■ ISF is 44 mg/dl. One unit of short-acting insulin decreases glucose by 44 mg/dl. It may be easier to round up to 45 or 50 mg/dl.

Another method of calculating an ISF is to use the general "safe" starting point of 50 mg/dl, i.e., 1 unit of rapid- or short-acting insulin decreases blood glucose by about 50 mg/dl. This method may work well for most lean-to-average adults. You may want to implement an ISF of 75 mg/dl for insulin-sensitive patients and an ISF of 100 mg/dl for children. Trial and error with meticulous record keeping will help determine a patient's specific ISF.

Once a person's ISF is calculated, multiplying it by 0.33 provides an insulin-to-carbohydrate ratio.

Example

■ ISF is 55 mg/dl

■ $55 \times 0.33 = 18.15$ (round to 18)

■ Insulin-to-carbohydrate ratio is 1:18

■ 1 unit of insulin covers 18 g carbohydrate

The ratios derived by any one of these three methods are merely starting points. Some clinicians begin by assuming an insulin-to-carbohydrate ratio of 1:15 for most lean-to-average adults, 1:10 ratio for insulin-resistant or overweight adults, and a ratio of 1:20 or 1:25 for most children, who tend to be more insulin sensitive.

After the insulin-to-carbohydrate ratio(s) and ISF have been established, meal and snack bolus doses can be calculated. You may want to provide written examples for the patient to review and, along with his or her ratio(s) and ISF, use to practice.

Example

■ Glucose target is 110 mg/dl

■ Insulin-to-carbohydrate ratio is 1:15

■ ISF is 50 mg/dl

■ Prelunch glucose is 187 mg/dl

Item	Carbohydrate (g)
1 turkey sandwich on rye bread	30
1 medium apple	25
8 oz 1% milk	12
Total	67

- Insulin needed to cover carbohydrate in meal is $67 \div 15 = 4.46$ units (round to 4.5)
- Insulin needed to return 187 mg/dl glucose to target is $187 - 110 = 77$ mg/dl over target $\div 50 = 1.54$ units (round to 1.5)
- $4.5 + 1.5$ for total premeal bolus of 6.0 units

Example

- Glucose target is 100 mg/dl
- Insulin-to-carbohydrate ratio is 1:18
- ISF is 70 mg/dl
- Predinner glucose is 204 mg/dl

Item	Carbohydrate (g)
3 oz baked chicken	0
½ cup mashed potatoes	15
1 dinner roll	15
1 cup tossed salad	(5; do not need to count)
½ cup broccoli	5
2 Tbsp salad dressing	(1; do not need to count)
½ cup fresh pineapple chunks	15
Total	50

- Insulin needed to cover carbohydrate in meal is $50 \div 18 = 2.77$ units (round to 2.8)
- Insulin needed to return 204 mg/dl glucose to target is $204 - 100 = 104$ mg/dl over target $\div 70 = 1.48$ units (round to 1.5)
- $2.8 + 1.5$ for total premeal bolus of 4.3 units

Detailed records of SMBG results, carbohydrate intake, and insulin doses provide useful information to make ratio adjustments. Some patients may need different ratios for different times of the day, but this is best determined after the basal rates are correctly calculated and fine-tuned. Remind patients to recalculate their insulin-to-carbohydrate ratio if:

- Total daily dose of insulin changes more than a few units
- Body weight changes more than a few pounds
- There are lifestyle changes, such as exercise, stress, work hours, illness, or pregnancy

IDENTIFYING AND MANAGING HYPERGLYCEMIA

Hyperglycemia can be troublesome, i.e., out-of-target values, or severe enough to cause DKA. Discuss with the patient what hyperglycemic values necessitate an insulin adjustment and what situation constitutes a hyperglycemic crisis.

If the patient experiences hyperglycemia, the first step is to eliminate the possibility of any technical problems with the pump. Each insulin pump manufacturer provides basic guidelines for troubleshooting the technical aspects and functions of the pump that can lead to hyperglycemia, including, but not limited, to:

- Loose Luer-lock connections
- Cracked infusion set tubing
- Dislodged infusion set
- Site irritation or infection
- Empty pump cartridge/reservoir
- Expired or spoiled insulin
- Incorrect bolus calculation
- Missed bolus doses
- Incorrectly programmed basal rates

Note that infusion tubing is double-layered and has an inner core that carries the insulin. Even tying knots in the tubing will not impede the insulin flow.

If the pump is functioning properly, then the patient must correct the hyperglycemia with a dose of insulin. To calculate the amount of insulin needed to return blood glucose to within the desired target range, patients need to know three factors:

- Their target level
- How much their glucose is above the target level
- Their ISF (for ISF calculations, see pages 23–25).

Example
- Target glucose level is 100 mg/dl
- Glucose is 264 mg/dl
- 264 mg/dl – 100 mg/dl = 164 mg/dl above target level
- ISF is 55 mg/dl
- 164 mg/dl ÷ 55 mg/dl = 2.9 units
- The correction dose of insulin is 2.9 units using an insulin pump (3 units if using a syringe or insulin pen)

If a correction is needed just before a meal, teach the patient to add the amount of insulin calculated for the correction dose to the amount of insulin needed to cover the carbohydrate he or she is about to eat.

Example
First, calculate the correction dose:
- Premeal glucose level is 226 mg/dl
- Target glucose level is 100 mg/dl
- 226 mg/dl – 100 mg/dl = 126 mg/dl
- ISF is 55 mg/dl
- 126 mg/dl ÷ 55 mg/dl = 2.3 units insulin to decrease the high premeal glucose level

Next, calculate the dose needed to cover the meal:
- 60 g carbohydrate are to be consumed
- Insulin-to-carbohydrate ratio is 1:15
- 60 ÷ 15 = 4 units insulin to cover the carbohydrate

Then, add the two doses together:
- 4 units + 2.3 units = 6.3 units insulin (insulin pump bolus) or round down to 6 units insulin if using syringe or pen

It is important that the high blood glucose level being corrected to premeal target range is actually the premeal blood glucose and not a glucose measurement taken 1–2 h after the last meal. A blood glucose measurement 1–2 h after a meal reflects the action of the previous pre-meal dose of rapid- or short-acting insulin, which is not yet complete. If a PPG result is used to calculate a correction dose, the insulin bolus doses may overlap and lead to postprandial hypoglycemia. Encourage pump patients to space meals at least 3–4 h apart and to make sure the dose they are calculating is based on the true premeal blood glucose. Provide instructions regarding specific insulin dose correction times.

Some clinicians prefer to have patients correct hyperglycemia using an algorithm. With this method, the patient calculates a PPG correction dose beginning with the preprandial glucose/PPG target. For example: bolus 1 unit of insulin for every 50 mg over 160 mg/dl at 3–4 h after eating. Other clinicians provide a sliding scale, e.g., bolus 1 unit if blood glucose is 150–200 mg/dl, bolus 2 units if glucose is 200–250 mg/dl. These algorithm methods result in corrections that are not as precise as those calculated using a specific ISF; they also re-quire the patient to memorize their algorithm list or carry it with them at all times. Pump therapy provides an opportunity to be more exact with insulin dosage. Patients may also find it easier to remember that "1 unit of insulin lowers my blood glucose ___ mg/dl" and to calculate an insulin dose using their individual ISF.

Another important issue in the management of hyperglycemia is the use of ketone test strips. Ask the patient to buy blood or urine ketone test strips, make sure the strips have not passed the expiration date, and know when and how to use them. Although ketone test strips are available over-the-counter, your patient may request or require a prescription for insurance reimbursement. Blood ketone strips require a meter.

Repeated episodes or a pattern of hyperglycemia require adjusting the basal rate(s), insulin-to-carbohydrate ratio, or ISF.

MANAGING HYPOGLYCEMIA

Hypoglycemia may be considered a downside of pump therapy. Because blood glucose is kept much closer to target, whether by MDI or insulin pump therapy, there is less of a "glucose buffer" against hypoglycemia. However, many studies reveal insulin pump therapy is associated with a marked decrease in the incidence of severe hypoglycemia from that seen during MDI therapy.[3,13,14] Insulin pump therapy is also beneficial is establishing and maintaining normoglycemia, and evidence indicates normoglycemia unequivocally decreases the development of hypoglycemia unawareness.[15,16]

Education on hypoglycemia management includes a review of basic guidelines, a glucagon prescription, and instructions on using glucagon for the patient's family members, friends, and significant other. This information should not be new to the patient or to the people around him or her. For mild to moderate hypoglycemia, teach and emphasize the Rule of 15:

- Treat hypoglycemia with 15 g fast-acting carbohydrate
- Check blood glucose after 15 min
- Repeat the treatment as needed

Remind the patient that overtreatment may create a vicious cycle of low blood glucose, high blood glucose, bolus doses, etc., with potential for subsequent weight gain. A general rule of thumb is that three or more unexplained instances of hypoglycemia in a week should prompt adjustments in basal rate(s), insulin-to-carbohydrate ratios, ISF, or a combination of these factors.

INFUSION SETS

Infusion sets distributed by the various pump and pump supply manufacturers may be interchangeable to work with several different brands of pumps. It is best to check with each pump company for specific guidelines. Although many brands exist, there are basically two types of infusion sets: metal needle and Teflon catheter or cannula. Metal needle infusion sets are usually less costly than the Teflon cannula sets, and both types are available in various models. The sets are inserted subcutaneously and the set "base" is attached to the insertion site with adhesive dressing or tape. An infusion set is worn for 2–3 days and then removed and discarded. Infusion sets left in longer lead to infection and/or scarring, which slows insulin delivery.

A metal needle infusion set requires that the needle stay under the skin and that the insertion base and tubing be attached to the site with either self-adhesive or separate dressing or tape. At present, medal needle infusion sets do not disconnect, although manufacturers may soon release ones that do. A variety of needles are available by type (straight or bent) and length (ranging from 8 to 16 mm). Children and lean adults may need shorter needles, whereas heavier people or large adults may need longer needles to guarantee subcutaneous insertion and placement. Some people find the metal needle sets to be uncomfortable because the needle may "pinch" or be felt during physical activity or movement. Many patients do not regard this as a deterrent to using this type of set. A major advantage of the metal needle infusion set is the guarantee of insulin delivery, as a metal needle cannot kink below the skin like a Teflon cannula set.

A Teflon cannula set uses a needle that is threaded into the cannula for subcutaneous insertion. After insertion, the needle is removed, leaving only the cannula below the skin and the infusion set base at the site. These set bases have self-adhesive tape or dressing. Some people find the length of a cannula infusion set needle intimidating and require reassurance and practice in insertion. A cannula set is more comfortable to wear than a metal needle set because the patient cannot feel the set when bending, twisting, or exercising. Teflon cannula sets may be straight or angled and come in different lengths. They also may include an optional handheld device to facilitate insertion of the needle.

Teflon cannula sets can disconnect at the site, providing greater lifestyle comfort and flexibility. The user unclips the tubing from the set base, leaving only the base and subcutaneous cannula in place, while removing the tubing, or most of it, and the pump. Some disconnect sets are self-sealing at the time of disconnection, whereas others require covers at the site as well as the end of the tubing. Teflon cannula sets cost at least 50% more than metal needle sets.

Discuss the features and benefits of each type of set with your patient (Table 3). Most people who use them enjoy the convenience of sets that disconnect. However, long-term pump users will often continue using their metal needle sets. Some patients use both types of sets and alternate depending on their activity.

Infusion set come in lengths ranging from 23 to 43 inches, depending on the manufacturer and the set. Manufacturers usually offer two or three tubing length options. Patients choose tubing length depending on their physical activity, sleeping habits, and clothing. For example, restless sleepers and people who wear their pump in their sock need longer tubing; those who wear the pump at their waist may prefer shorter tubing. Any excess tubing can be easily tucked into the patient's clothing and kept out of sight. Tying the tubing in knots does not impede the delivery of insulin.

Infusion Set Insertion

The patient may have already observed the insertion and removal of an infusion set when deciding whether or not to try pump therapy (see Chapter 2). If not, the patient should see a demonstration now, especially if he or she is anxious about inserting or wearing an infusion set. During pump start-up, the patient will learn how to prepare the skin and insert the infusion set. Pump manufacturer personnel also provide specific instructions and detailed information to pump patients about infusion set insertion procedures.

The abdomen is the preferred infusion site because it offers a consistent rate of absorption. However, pump patients have had success using other subcutaneous sites, e.g., the upper hip/buttock, thigh, and

TABLE 3. Comparison of Features in Both Types of Infusion Sets

Feature	Metal needle	Teflon cannula
Needle is removed after insertion	No	Yes
Can disconnect for bathing, intimacy	No	Yes
Set felt while bending or engaging in some physical activity?	Yes	No
Risk of insulin nondelivery from set kinking under the skin	Low	Higher

upper arm. Avoid inserting the set within a 2-inch diameter of the navel, at the waistline or belt area, or in any area where clothing would rub against or constrict the site.

Infusion sets must be changed every 2–3 days to prevent infection and scar tissue buildup, which can lead to occlusions and reduce or interrupt delivery of insulin. The site should be rotated every time the infusion set is replaced, usually from one side of the body to the other, and 1/2 to 1 inch away from a previous site. The patient must check the site at least once daily for redness, tenderness, and tape or dressing placement.

Steps for infusion set insertion:

1. Wash hands with antibacterial soap.
2. Assemble the infusion set supplies in a well-lit, clean workspace.
3. Prepare the infusion site using an antibacterial soap or solution or a commercial product, such as IV Prep. Allow the skin to dry naturally. Anxious children and apprehensive adults may benefit from the use of a topical analgesic to numb the skin before inserting the infusion set.
4. Follow the manufacturer's instructions for the infusion set insertion and needle removal if using a cannula set.
5. Secure the set to the site with sterile dressing or tape.
6. If using a disconnect cannula set, follow the manufacturer's instructions to attach the tubing and bolus insulin to fill the cannula.

A metal needle set may be felt, whereas a Teflon cannula set will not. If a set becomes uncomfortable after it is in position, it should be removed and discarded, and a new one should be inserted in a different site. If the site becomes red, swollen, irritated, or painful, the patient should remove and discard the set and rotate the site. The set should also be changed if blood appears in the tubing.

OPTIONAL SALINE TRIAL

An optional saline trial can be done with a loaner pump while patients are deciding whether a pump is the right tool for them or after the pump is purchased and delivered during the pump preparation period. A saline trial may help the patient decide which pump to choose (see Chapter 3.) People who are unsure about "being attached to something 24 h a day" or have anxiety about infusion set insertion may find that wearing a pump with saline allays fears and concerns. A saline trial also provides the patient the opportunity to learn the functions of the pump (the "buttonology") without feeling the pressure of, "If I press this button, I might make a mistake." The insulin start that follows a saline trial may serve as a review of the technical training of the pump initiation process. This may be beneficial to those patients who are not quick learners or who express nervousness or anxiety about their actual pump start.

A saline trial should not be mandatory. MDI therapy must continue while wearing a saline pump; therefore, the patient does twice the work without enjoying the flexibility or freedom associated with pump therapy. And a patient who is excited about pump therapy is impatient to get started. A pump patient who is required by his or her clinician or CDE to wear the pump with saline first may resent the delay in the pump start and view it as a waste of time. The clinician and patient, or parents of the pediatric patient, should decide together if a saline start is truly appropriate. Saline requires a prescription, which the prescribing physician must provide to the patient.

LIFESTYLE ISSUES

Many prospective pump users hesitate or neglect to ask about lifestyle concerns; therefore, the health care professional must take the initiative and include this information in the pump education process.

Daily wear

The pump can be worn by several different means, including a clip, a case (leather, vinyl, or plastic) with or without a built-in clip or belt loops, or inside clothing such as thigh or leg garments, boxer shorts, lounging pants, and slips with pump pouches or pockets. A cotton infant sock is another option: the pump fits into the sock easily and can be worn in the side or cup of a bra, under control-top pantyhose, or pinned inside clothing. Some patients wear the pump in the top of their sock with long infusion set tubing under their pants and use an audio or remote feature to deliver bolus insulin as needed. Another option is to sew pockets into the seams of garments or use Velcro for removable pockets. Ask the pump patient in training to plan ahead on how to wear the pump with various types of clothing.

Sleeping

Every new pump user wonders what to do with his or her pump during sleep. The patient may want to try wearing the pump inside the pocket of pajamas, a nightshirt, a nightgown, or boxer shorts. Another option is placing the pump in a specific location, such as under the pillow or on a night table. The pump can also be clipped to a sheet or blanket or placed freely in the bed. Longer tubing provides greater flexibility for moving and turning. Reassure the pump patient that even if the tubing is knotted upon awakening, insulin delivery will not be disturbed. The infusion set dressing or tape secures the infusion set safely to the site.

Use of an electric blanket can affect the potency of insulin, especially if the pump is directly on the heating coils. Pump users need to consider this if their fasting blood glucose is erratic without explanation.   ·

Bathing/showering

Some pumps are waterproof or water resistant—check with the pump manufacturer for specific guidelines. Even if the pump patient is not planning on wearing the pump while bathing or showering, pumps have been known to fall in the toilet. With a disconnect infusion set, the pump can be disconnected for up to 1 h and reconnected after bathing or showering. A metal needle (nondisconnect) infusion set requires a waterproof or water-resistant pump, or the patient must remove and discard the set and insert a new one after the bath or shower. Remind the patient that insulin is very heat sensitive; soaking in a hot bath or whirlpool or using a sauna while wearing the pump is not recommended.

Intimacy

To wear the pump or not during intimacy is the patient's choice. If the patient wants to keep the pump connected, longer infusion set tubing is recommended. Also, a decreased basal rate may be necessary for a few hours. The infusion site should always be checked to make certain the set has remained intact.

The pump user who temporarily disconnects his or her infusion set may want to deliver a compensatory bolus before removing the pump. For example, if the basal rate is 0.6 units/h and the pump will be removed for 1.5 h, the compensatory bolus would be 0.9 units delivered before disconnecting or removing the pump. Remind the patient that increased physical activity may necessitate a decreased amount of insulin and that trial and error will determine this information. The patient should be reminded to reconnect his or her infusion set.

Managing sick days and medical procedures

The pump patient uses the same basic sick day guidelines that apply to anyone using insulin:

- Check and record the results of blood glucose more frequently.
- If blood glucose exceeds 240 mg/dl on two occasions, check ketones.
- Do not decrease basal insulin doses; basal rates may need to be increased 20–50% for the duration of the illness. Mild colds, the flu, and dental surgery may require smaller temporary increases (10–20%) or other adjustments in basal rates.
- Increase noncaloric fluids.
- If lack of appetite or vomiting exists, substitute caloric/carbohydrate-containing fluids for solid foods, if tolerated.
- Call physician or appropriate health care professional if hyperglycemia, nausea, vomiting, or diarrhea persists for >4 h; if there is a fever >100°; or if there are moderate to large ketones present in the urine.

Patients should know how to program their pump for temporary rate changes. Remind the patient that if basal rates are set correctly, the omission of food should not result in hypoglycemia. On the contrary, hyperglycemia may occur rapidly during illness and, if untreated, lead to ketosis and ketoacidosis. Go over the patient's plan of action for severe illness or emergency. (Pump manufacturer customer support staff cannot provide medical treatment guidelines for insulin pump therapy patients.)

During hospitalization, pump therapy is at the discretion of the admitting physician and may require limited staff training. Some hospitals have protocols for the admission of insulin pump therapy patients. Psychiatric admissions may necessitate removal of the pump and a return to injection therapy monitored and administered by the hospital staff.

For outpatient procedures and surgeries, pump therapy is usually continued, and the patient and/or the health care team must provide basic information to the procedure or surgical staff team. This information may include the need to tape or secure the pump to the hospital gown, what to do or whom to call if the pump alarm sounds during the procedure, and an alternative insulin delivery plan if the pump must be removed. The patient should remove his or her pump during an MRI or CAT scan procedure. X-rays do not harm the pump, but the pump user may feel more comfortable removing the pump or placing it out of the range of the X-ray.

Exercise

Even at this advanced stage of diabetes education, many patients do not realize that exercise, depending on the type, intensity, and duration, can decrease blood glucose levels for up to 36 h. Nor do patients realize that strenuous exercise can increase the secretion of the stress hormones glucagon, cortisol, and epinephrine, resulting in an increase in blood glucose. The necessary detailed fine-tuning of basal rate and dietary intake adjustments can take several months after pump initiation. Until initial basal rates have been established, the new pump patient should omit moderate to strenuous exercise. The patient can resume planned exercise once he or she understands how to modify basal rates and carbohydrate intake to compensate for exercise. This requires detailed SMBG record keeping before, during, and after exercise, as well as noting dietary intake and insulin doses. Emphasize detailed record keeping to establish a pattern of appropriate adjustments.

In general, it is best to begin exercise when blood glucose is >100 and <150 mg/dl. The pump provides the option of adjusting basal rates before, during, and/or after exercise. Mild to moderate exercise requires a 10–30% decrease in basal rate during the exercise activity.[9] Some clinicians begin with a 25–50% decrease. A temporary basal rate should be implemented before and after, as well as during, the exercise or sport. The new temporary basal rate can begin 30–60 min before the exercise and may require continuance for several hours after, depending on the intensity and duration of the activity. Additional carbohydrate may be necessary to prevent hypoglycemia. Table 4 provides some starting points for these adjustments.

If the patient chooses to wear the pump during sports or exercise, it can be securely attached with a clip or case. Some cases have a hard plastic insert or exterior to provide additional protection to the pump during contact sports. The tubing can be anchored down with additional tape or dressing as needed. At present, waterproof pumps can be used in depths ranging from 8 to 12 feet for varying periods of time without any problem. The pump manufacturer can provide specifics on waterproof or water-resistant capabilities.

TABLE 4. Suggested Basal Rate and Carbohydrate Intake
Modifications for Various Levels of Exercise

Level of activity	Basal rate decrease (%)	Additional carbohydrate/ hour (g)
Mild (walking, gardening)	10	7–15
Moderate (biking, golf/walking)	30	15
Strenuous (jogging, soccer)	50	15–30
Sustained activity over a few days (hiking, skiing, or rowing)	20–30	±15 (varies)

Adapted from Kaufman et al.[9]

The pump is generally removed for contact sports or strenuous
exercise or water activity, such as water skiing. A disconnectable infusion set makes this convenient and may be self-sealing or have covers
for sealing the end of the tubing and the infusion site base. Individuals
using a metal needle (nondisconnect) infusion set must discard the
infusion set and insert a new set at the end of the activity. It is generally recommended to not suspend the pump during a brief disconnection period. Allowing the pump to deliver the basal rate while
disconnected from the user can prevent the development of a clog at
the end of the infusion set tubing.

Because of the short action and duration of rapid- and short-
acting insulin, the pump should not be disconnected for more than
1 h. If necessary, the pump user can calculate the percent change in
basal rate and deliver the reduced hourly basal rate in the form of a
bolus. Again, individualization is essential and requires trial and error
fine-tuning.

Worst case scenario survival

Prepare your patients to deal with the worst possible situation. Pump
users have been mugged and had their pump stolen because it was
mistaken for a cell phone or beeper. Pumps have fallen off while the
patient was closing the car door, leaving the infusion set attached to
the body but cut by the car door, with the pump left on the road.
Physical activity, excessive perspiration, unplanned exposure to
water, and even clothes shopping can dislodge or cause accidental removal of the infusion set. A dropped pump can break. A malfunc-
tioning pump or even a severe infusion site infection constitutes an
emergency.

People who wear insulin pumps must be prepared at all times with a backup system to continue insulin delivery. Pump patients no longer have intermediate- or long-acting insulin to protect them from the rapid onset of ketosis or ketoacidosis.

All people with diabetes should wear some form of medical identification. A pump patient's medical identification should indicate "on insulin pump" or "uses insulin pump." Suggested items to carry at **all** times include:

- Treatment for hypoglycemia
- Glucose meter, lancets, meter batteries, and strips or sensors
- Infusion set(s)
- Skin prep pad or other site preparation supplies
- Alcohol swab
- Site dressing or tape
- Insulin pen with rapid- or short-acting insulin *or* rapid- or short-acting insulin vial to fill pump cartridge/reservoir
- Syringe for injection *or* insulin pen with rapid- or short-acting insulin
- Rapid- or short-acting insulin vial for syringe or pump cartridge/reservoir
- Pump batteries and insertion/removal tools, if necessary
- Physician name, address, and phone numbers
- Emergency contact addresses and phone numbers

Travel

Traveling takes even more foresight and planning on the part of the pump patient. The upside is that an insulin pump makes travel easier and more enjoyable. In addition to packing daily supplies, plus 50% more for emergencies or delayed return, advise the patient to have:

- Spare pump, if available
- Spare glucose meter and supplies, if available
- Additional treatment for hypoglycemia
- Container for used lancets and infusion sets
- Ketone check strips
- Glucagon treatment, which travel partner(s) should know how to use
- Intermediate- or long-acting insulin in original box with prescription label
- Copy of prepump or appropriate injection therapy regimen
- Prescriptions for insulin, pump supplies, and other medications

This information was supplied to the American Diabetes Association from the Federal Aviation Administration (FAA) regarding people with diabetes flying within the 50 United States:

- Passengers may board with syringes or insulin delivery systems if accompanied by the insulin in its original pharmaceutically labeled box. No exceptions will be made.
- Passengers who test glucose but do not require insulin may board with their capped lancets if accompanied by a glucose meter that has the manufacturer's name embossed on the meter.
- Passengers can carry on a glucagon kit intact in its original preprinted pharmaceutically labeled container.
- **Prescriptions and letters of medical necessity will not be accepted.**
- Passengers should call the airline carrier at least 1 day in advance of a scheduled flight to confirm what that airline's policy is with regard to diabetes medication and supplies. Be advised that each airline's policy is subject to change.
- Passengers with disabilities should expect nondiscriminatory treatment as required by the Air Carrier Access Act (ACAA). A passenger encountering any diabetes-related difficulty because of security measures should ask to speak with a Complaints Resolution Official (CRO) for the airline. Each airline must provide a CRO who is entitled to act on behalf of the airline in ACAA cases.

- Letter from prescribing physician stating patient uses pump therapy and is required to carry listed items
- Extra prescription eyeglasses
- Name, address, and phone number of physician/medical personnel at destination location

All travel items should be packed in carry-on luggage, and, if possible, divided between travel partners. Automobile, train, and airline travel may require refrigeration of insulin, depending on the length of the trip and storage conditions.

An insulin pump may be detected at security checkpoints, depending on the sensitivity of the security system. Most rail and airline security personnel are familiar with an insulin pump but may require the patient to show the pump and corresponding letter and prescription from the physician.

When changing time zones, it is best to keep the pump on local time while traveling and reset the pump clock upon arrival at the new destination. For time changes of 1 h, it may not be necessary to make basal rate adjustments. Time zone changes of >3 h may require a gradual change in resetting the pump clock, e.g., 1–2 h each day, to better match the body's diurnal clock change. Bolus doses should be administered as usual, and frequent SMBG is required.

CHAPTER 5

Pump Start-Up

PUMP START BASICS

Typically, the pump start-up education session takes 2–4 h and requires the undivided attention of the pump user or parent(s). Pump training can be done in an outpatient setting, such as the clinician's office or the patient's home, with permission and approval of the prescribing physician. Inpatient admissions are usually no longer required by insurance companies but may be desired by either the clinician or patient. An inpatient admission is usually for one overnight stay, allowing close monitoring of nocturnal and fasting blood glucose levels, and may be most beneficial for children. Another option is the "23-h observational stay," i.e., the patient is trained, monitored, and discharged 1 h short of a 24-h stay, thus avoiding charges for and a record of a hospital admission.

Carefully set the pump start-up date. Make sure that the first few weeks of pump therapy are fairly routine, and avoid situations or conditions that may adversely affect blood glucose levels or interfere with the establishment of basal rates, such as:

- Menstruation, and a few days before menstruation
- Out-of-town or unusual travel
- Unusual work, school, or leisure-activity schedules

- Moderate-to-strenuous exercise, including major sports activities
- Outpatient surgery, including dental work
- Holidays
- Limited access to telephone and/or fax communication

Pump start-up orders must be provided to the patient several days in advance. Most endocrinologists and CDEs use forms to provide instructions for "weaning" the patient off intermediate- or long-acting insulin. Other written instructions for the patient include blood glucose monitoring and dietary guidelines, a list of supplies to bring to the pump start-up appointment, and specific information regarding appointment time and location (see Appendixes).

Because the pump start is best initiated without the interference of any lasting effect of intermediate- or long-acting insulin, the start is usually scheduled in the morning after the patient has taken his or her rapid- or fast-acting insulin to cover the breakfast meal. The last dose of intermediate insulin (NPH or lente) should be administered at least 12 h before the scheduled pump start (12–18 h recommended). The bedtime dose can be given as usual the evening before the pump start because the actual "hook up" to the pump occurs at the end of the start-up training period late the next morning. The patient should administer the last dose of long-acting insulin at least 24 h in advance (24–48 h recommended). Some clinicians choose to continue the long-acting insulin and decrease the dose by 50% the day preceding the pump start and/or initiate a reduced starting pump basal rate. Another option is to discontinue the ultralente or glargine insulin 24–36 h in advance of the pump start, substituting calculated doses of intermediate-acting insulin, with the last dose being administered the evening before the pump start. Do not discontinue intermediate- or long-acting insulin and substitute with multiple doses of rapid-acting insulin every 3–4 h throughout the night before the pump start. The result will be a tired and "out-of-sorts" patient whose sleep has been disrupted.

PUMP START GUIDELINES FOR THE PATIENT

On the pump start day, the patient should:

1. Eat a usual breakfast, following appropriate rapid- or short-acting insulin injection.

2. Wear comfortable two-piece clothing, not dresses or one-piece garments.
3. Bring the following items:
   - **New** vial of prescribed rapid- or fast-acting insulin at room temperature; a partially used vial should **not** be used because the patient may have previously incorrectly mixed his or her rapid- or short-acting insulin with the intermediate- or long-acting insulin, and the vial may be contaminated with drops of the cloudy insulin.
   - Glucose meter, lancets, strips/sensors
   - Glucose log book
   - Hypoglycemia treatment
   - Target glycemic levels, insulin-to-carbohydrate ratio, and ISF
   - Calculator
   - Paper and pen
4. Come ready for a 3- to 4-h education session.

If the patient received the pump at home, he or she should check the box and match its contents with shipping information several days in advance of the pump start. Emphasize to the patient that he or she needs to bring the entire box with all contents to the pump start. Each pump shipment should contain:

- New pump (and spare, if appropriate)
- Batteries
- Syringes/cartridges
- Skin prep product(s)
- Infusion sets
- Infusion site dressings
- User's manual
- Instructional video and/or CD, if available
- Warranty card/information
- Additional written materials (e.g., accessory catalogs, special instructions)

PUMP START GUIDELINES FOR THE CLINICIAN

If the pump and corresponding supplies were shipped to the clinician's site, open the box and inspect it for completeness several days preceding the pump start.

An insulin pump start-up training session includes a review of the pump, accessories, and instructions for use:

- Inserting and removing the batteries
- Filling and placing the pump insulin syringe/cartridge and lead screw, if applicable
- Attaching the infusion set tubing to the pump
- Priming the tubing, i.e., filling the infusion set with insulin
- Programming the pump ("buttonology" training) and setting all applicable features, such as clock, date, sound volume, language, basal rates, bolus increments, bolus deliveries, temporary basal settings, memory, and pump suspension; reviewing waterproof specifics
- Delivering a bolus into midair for practice
- Stopping a bolus mid-delivery
- Recognizing and acting on any warnings or alarms
- Preparing the infusion site
- Inserting the infusion set, using insertion device, if applicable
- Inspecting the infusion set
- Discussing the troubleshooting guidelines, i.e., reviewing technical problems that can occur with the pump and/or infusion site and set, such as site tenderness, tubing leakage, or air bubbles in tubing
- Reviewing the user's manual and completing the pump warranty information
- Reviewing of any other accompanying pump manufacturer literature, including accessory catalogs, specific instructions, or technical changes that do not appear in the user's manual
- Identifying the contact names and numbers of pump manufacturer representatives or customer service for technical assistance
- Reviewing follow-up and management guidelines as outlined by the prescribing physician, including target glycemic levels, insulin-to-carbohydrate ratio, ISF, and contact names and numbers
- Completing pump training checklist with copies provided to the pump manufacturer, prescribing physician, and CDE

The clinician is responsible for providing pump start orders to the educator providing the pump start-up training. These include:

- Starting basal rate(s)
- Insulin-to-carbohydrate ratio(s)

■ ISF and instructions for use (may delay implementation until basal rates have been fine-tuned)
■ SMBG instructions
■ Communication guidelines, i.e., who, when, and where does the patient call for reporting SMBG results and technical assistance

DETERMINING STARTING BASAL RATE

The basal rate is usually 40–50% of the total daily dose (TDD), with the remainder comprised of bolus insulin doses. Insulin-resistant and adolescent patients and patients with type 2 diabetes may require higher basal amounts. Some clinicians use 45–60% of the TDD as basal insulin.[6] Generally, the basal rate should be no more than 60% of the patient's TDD. If the patient's recent glycemic control has been within desired target ranges, the TDD may need to be reduced 10–25% because most people require less insulin with pump therapy.

There are several methods for determining starting basal rate. Unless the clinician is certain of the exact hours the patient experiences either surges or decreases in blood glucose levels, **it is best to initiate pump therapy with one basal rate**, and make changes as needed. Pump therapy initiation often reveals blood glucose increases due to the dawn phenomenon and blood glucose reductions that differ in timing from what may have been assumed on MDI therapy.

Method 1
1. Determine the patient's TDD by adding all doses of rapid- or short-acting and intermediate- or long-acting insulin together.
2. Calculate 40% of the TDD and divide by 24. This calculation yields an hourly starting basal rate (J.H. Mersey, K.M. Bolderman, unpublished data).

Example
1. TDD: 34 units (5 units aspart before breakfast and before evening meal + 10 units a.m. NPH + 14 units hs NPH = 34 units total)
2. 34 units × 0.4 = 13.6 units ÷ 24 h = 0.56. The starting basal rate is 0.5 units/h (or 0.55 units/h if pump can be programmed in twentieth-unit increments) × 24 h.

Method 2

1. Determine the patient's TDD by adding all doses of rapid- or short-acting and intermediate- or long-acting insulin together.
2. Calculate 75–90% of the TDD. Use one-half of this amount and divide by 24. This calculation yields an hourly starting basal rate.

Example 1

1. TDD: 34 units (5 units aspart before breakfast and before evening meal + 10 units a.m. NPH + 14 units hs NPH = 34 units total)
2. 34 units × 0.75 = 25.5 units ÷ 2 = 12.75 ÷ 24 h = 0.53. The starting basal rate is 0.5 units/h (or 0.55 units/h if pump can be programmed in twentieth-unit increments) × 24 h.

Example 2

1. TDD: 34 units (5 units aspart before breakfast and before evening meal + 10 units a.m. NPH + 14 units hs NPH = 34 units total)
2. 34 units × 0.90 = 30.6 units ÷ 2 = 15.3 ÷ 24 h = 0.64. The starting basal rate is 0.6 units/h (or 0.65 units/h if pump can be programmed in twentieth-unit increments × 24 h.

Method 3

1. If using multiple doses of rapid- or short-acting insulin with one dose of glargine, use the dose of glargine as the basal dose for the pump.
2. Divide the total dose of glargine by 24. This calculation yields an hourly starting basal rate.

Example

1. Dose of glargine = 20 units.
2. 20 units ÷ 24 h = 0.83. Starting basal rate is 0.8 or 0.85 units/h × 24 h.

Be conservative in implementing the starting rate if recent glucose records reveal frequent hypoglycemia. Initiate a rate slightly lower (by 0.1 or 0.05) than what was calculated. Increase the calculated rate slightly if recent blood glucose levels have been consistently elevated (>200 mg/dl). One leveling technique is to calculate starting basal rates using more than one method. Results are compared and averaged, or the lowest basal rate calculated is used.

FOLLOW-UP INSTRUCTIONS

The patient should perform a glucose check and administer a bolus, if necessary, to correct hyperglycemia at the end of the pump start-up training. The prescribing physician and/or CDE should give the patient specific instructions for follow-up and management during the first few weeks after pump start-up (see Appendixes). These include:

- Perform SMBG a minimum of six times per day (3:00 a.m., fasting, before each meal, and bedtime) and record results. Additional postprandial checks at 2–3 h are also useful, and many patients actually add these tests to their regimen. If, after a few days, a dawn phenomenon is detected and a compensatory basal rate adjustment is made and verified, the 3:00 a.m. check becomes unnecessary.
- Record grams of carbohydrate consumed and specific foods and beverages. This routine is especially helpful in identifying correct meal and snack bolus doses.
- Avoid alcohol; high-fat foods, such as pizza, cakes, pies, some snack products, and some ethnic meals, including Italian, Mexican, and Chinese; and foods not usually consumed. Remind the patient to stick with a "basic" diet or "plain foods" and eliminate any food that could adversely cause erratic glucose levels.
- Avoid moderate to strenuous exercise.
- Record all bolus doses using the insulin-to-carbohydrate ratio for meals and snacks and any ISF bolus doses given for hyperglycemia. It may be best to delay use of the ISF until the basal rates have been established because a correction bolus can lower blood glucose readings. If the correct basal rates have not been established, the clinician will not know if the basal insulin or the bolus dose is causing glucose fluctuations. The ISF dose should always be delivered if the patient is symptomatically hyperglycemic.
- Record any unexpected or unusual events that could affect blood glucose levels, e.g., stress or illness.
- Call in, fax, or e-mail the information to the clinician/CDE **daily**. Provide specific names, numbers, and times to reach the clinician/CDE. Call the clinician/CDE for assistance with glycemic control or illness.
- Call the pump manufacturer with any questions or problems related to the technical functions of the pump.

A patient may require a follow-up visit within 1 week to review and observe an infusion set site change and pump syringe/cartridge removal and new fill. Some clinicians/CDEs do this "as needed," whereas others schedule an automatic 1-week brief appointment. Family support is critical in the first few weeks after pump start-up, and including the new pump patient's family members and significant other in a meeting to review lifestyle issues during this time may be helpful.

The patient should schedule a return visit to the clinician 4–6 weeks after the pump start-up for a review of SMBG and insulin doses and inspection of infusion sites. Many patients feel empowered after initiating pump therapy and will delay or reschedule appointments with their physician and/or CDEs, saying, "I'm doing great on the pump. I don't need to see my doctor or educator right now." Although self-management at the highest levels of diabetes care is the goal, emphasize to the patient the importance of clinical monitoring of A1C quarterly (patients with type 1 diabetes) or biannually (patients with type 2 diabetes) and good communication with the health care team. Ask the pump patient to maintain a regular visit/appointment schedule with health care providers to evaluate his or her level of control, glucose patterns, insulin doses, and the pump's features and options. An insulin pump is a wonderful diabetes management tool, but it is not a license for the patient to practice medicine.

CHAPTER 6

Pump
Management

Patients are "fine-tuned" when the basal rate(s) and bolus doses, determined using the insulin-to-carbohydrate ratio and ISF, yield results within the patient's target glycemic levels. This outcome takes a minimum of several weeks or longer. The patient needs to collect information, e.g., SMBG records, carbohydrate intake, and bolus doses, to assist the clinician in evaluating his or her status. Careful monitoring and detailed record keeping in the early stages of pump therapy, although tedious, are necessary and beneficial.

The management of pump therapy requires assessing, evaluating, and modifying the basal rates, insulin-to-carbohydrate ratios, and ISF. When making changes with the patient, explain why and how adjustments are made. Your explanations will help increase the patient's understanding of the basics of pump therapy and build confidence in his or her ability to identify problems and practice appropriate self-management pump skills.

Once the initial basal rates and insulin doses have been determined, the patient and health care team can continue to tailor the pump therapy. Different basal rates, insulin-to-carbohydrate ratios, and ISFs to accommodate such normal events as exercise, stress, and the menstrual cycle can be established. Taking pump therapy to this next level requires additional detailed monitoring, record keeping, and trial and error but is worthwhile.

ADJUSTING BASAL RATE

The underlying cause of erratic glucose readings is usually an incorrect basal rate(s). However, do not make any basal rate changes in the first 24 h after pump start-up unless there is a blatant need, such as repeated or severe hypoglycemia or hyperglycemia. Hypoglycemia may be due to the lingering effects of intermediate- or long-acting insulin. Also, the new pump user is commonly anxious for the first day or two; making changes in the initial basal rate or adding a second rate may be premature.

The first step in dealing with out-of-target glucose levels is to check and correct the basal rate(s). Changing the insulin-to-carbohydrate ratio or ISF before correcting the basal rate(s) will not necessarily solve the problem of erratic glucose readings. The basal rate(s) is correct if the patient can skip or delay meals and 3- or 4-h PPG readings fall within target, not varying by >30 mg/dl from the premeal glucose level. Explain the goal of establishing appropriate basal rates to the patient this way: "If you were to fast for 24 h and did not have or do anything to affect your glucose level, such as food, exercise, stress, illness, or hormonal changes, your basal rates should not let your glucose readings vary by more than 30 mg/dl throughout the entire 24 h." The 3:00 a.m. and fasting blood glucose readings should be within 30 mg/dl of the previous day's bedtime glucose reading. This is the goal when checking basal rates.

To check basal rates, first fix the fasting glucose. Ask the patient to:

1. Check and record the bedtime glucose reading. Do not correct it. If the bedtime glucose has been consistently <70 mg/dl or >240 mg/dl, decrease or increase the pre-evening meal bolus before performing the basal rate check again. The patient should always treat for hypoglycemia.

2. Check and record the 3:00 a.m. glucose reading. If hypoglycemic, treat. You may need to decrease the basal rate that covers bedtime to 3:00 a.m. Do not correct for a 3:00 a.m. hyperglycemic reading unless the patient is symptomatic or has a glucose reading >240 mg/dl.

3. Check and record the fasting glucose level.

4. Compare the three readings. Increase or decrease the basal rate by 0.05 or 0.10 beginning at the time of the last glucose check preceding the glucose elevation.

Example

- Basal rate is 0.8 units/h × 24 h
- 4-h postprandial bedtime glucose at 11:00 p.m. is 186 mg/dl
- 3:00 a.m. glucose is 202 mg/dl

Solution: There are two possibilities. If the 7:45 a.m. fasting glucose is 248 mg/dl, this patient has a strong dawn phenomenon. A second and higher basal rate needs to be initiated at 3:00 a.m. to correct the elevated fasting glucose reading. Increase the 0.8 units/h rate to 0.9 units/h for the period from 3:00 to 8:00 a.m., and repeat the basal check test the next evening. Repeat and increase by 0.1-unit increments until the fasting glucose is within 30 mg/dl of the 3:00 a.m. reading. However, if the 7:45 a.m. fasting glucose is 197 mg/dl, a different basal rate from 11:00 p.m. to 8:00 a.m. is **not** needed because all three glucose readings are within the same range. Instead, the elevated bedtime glucose reading needs to be corrected. Either the early evening-to-bedtime basal rate needs to be increased or the insulin-to-carbohydrate ratio for the evening meal needs to be increased.

Once the fasting glucose is "fixed," additional basal rate checks may be needed to correct erratic daytime-to-bedtime glucose readings.

Basal rate checks require fasting and are best done in blocks of time versus a 24-h fast. Identify the postprandial period that requires alteration and choose the block of time to test, i.e., breakfast to lunch, lunch to dinner, or dinner to bedtime. To perform a basal rate check, ask the patient to choose a day free of influence of exercise, stress, menstrual hormone surges, etc.

1. Check and record a 2- to 4-h PPG level (premeal bolus given normally). Do not correct unless hypoglycemic.
2. Check and record glucose every 1–2 h for the next 4–6 h, or however long the patient is willing to fast.
3. Compare the results. If glucose has risen or fallen >30 mg/dl from the previous reading, the basal rate needs to be changed.
4. Implement a basal rate change in 0.05- or 0.1-unit increments beginning at the time preceding the last glucose rise or fall.

Example

- 7:00 a.m. to 4:00 p.m. basal rate is 0.6 units/h.
- FBG is 108 mg/dl, within target. Breakfast is at 7:00 a.m.
- 3-h breakfast (10:00 a.m.) PPG: 123 mg/dl

- 4-h breakfast (11:00 a.m.) PPG: 119 mg/dl
- Omit lunch.
- 5-h breakfast (12:00 p.m.) PPG: 148 mg/dl
- 6-h breakfast (1:00 p.m.) PPG: 192 mg/dl

Solution: An increase in the basal rate is needed starting at 11:00 a.m., which is 1 h before the first glucose elevation begins. Increase the basal rate to 0.7 units/h from 11:00 a.m. to 3:00 p.m. Ask the patient to perform another basal rate check a few days later beginning with lunch, i.e., the patient should eat lunch (with premeal bolus taken as normal) then check glucose hourly for 5–6 h afterward. Make adjustments in 0.05- or 0.1-unit increments as needed. The patient may need to perform basal rate checks over several days to determine appropriate 24-h rates.

For patients whose initial or corrected basal rates are >1.0 units/h, an increase or decrease in increments >0.1 unit may be indicated. A basal rate change should be between 10 and 20%. Be conservative.

ADJUSTING INSULIN-TO-CARBOHYDRATE RATIO

After the 24-h basal rates have been determined, the patient should continue to monitor and record intake, glucose, bolus doses, exercise, etc., for your review. If PPG readings are not within target, the insulin-to-carbohydrate ratio needs adjusting. This is common and takes time to correct.

To correct postprandial hyperglycemia, the patient needs more insulin to cover less carbohydrate. Adjust the insulin-to-carbohydrate ratio by 3–5 g carbohydrate.

Example
- Basal rates have been determined by basal check tests.
- Insulin-to-carbohydrate ratio is 1 unit:15 g. The patient counted carbohydrate and calculated meal bolus accurately and correctly.
- 3-h PPG is 210 mg/dl.

Solution: Decrease the insulin-to-carbohydrate ratio to 1:12, continue monitoring, and decrease the ratio as needed.

Postprandial hypoglycemia requires less insulin to cover carbohydrate.

Example
- Basal rates have been determined by basal check tests.
- Insulin-to-carbohydrate ratio is 1 unit:15 g. The patient counted carbohydrate and calculated meal bolus accurately and correctly.
- 3-h PPG is 72 mg/dl.

Solution: Increase the insulin-to-carbohydrate ratio to 1:20, continue monitoring, and change the ratio as needed.

Sometimes, patients require different ratios for different meals. Another consideration in reviewing the insulin-to-carbohydrate ratio and meal bolus is the use of a delayed bolus, i.e., extended bolus or square wave bolus. Spreading the bolus out over several hours may help prevent unexplained or troublesome postprandial hypoglycemia or hyperglycemia. Using a delayed bolus when eating pizza is a common practice to help correct the early postprandial hypoglycemia and a 5- to 6-h delayed hyperglycemia. A delayed bolus is also helpful for the patient who has gastroparesis or who consumes high-protein or high-fat foods, although this practice warrants additional research and a trial-and-error approach.

ADJUSTING INSULIN SENSITIVITY FACTOR

A correctly calculated ISF bolus allows an elevated postprandial blood glucose level to return to target within ~3–5 h. With rapid-acting insulin, the decrease may be noted within 3 h; it takes about 5 h with short-acting insulin. The patient should track the glucose level hourly for several hours after a correction bolus to determine the effectiveness of the ISF.

If the 3- to 5-h post-bolus glucose level is still elevated, the ISF needs to be increased.

Example
- John's 3-h PPG is 276 mg/dl. He realizes the premeal insulin bolus was too small for his meal and calculates a correction bolus according to his target and ISF.
- John's 3- to 4-h PPG target is 100 mg/dl and his ISF is 50 mg/dl.
- 276 – 100 = 176 mg/dl above target.
- 176 mg/dl ÷ 50 mg/dl = 3.52, so John's correction bolus is 3.5 units.

▨ John rechecks his glucose 3 h after the 3.5-unit bolus, and his glucose is 165 mg/dl, 65 mg/dl above his target. His ISF needs to be changed.

▨ Instead of using 1 unit to lower glucose by 50 mg/dl, John tries a new ISF of 40 mg/dl, i.e., 1 unit lowers his glucose 40 mg/dl.

Patients may need to try different ISFs before the correct ISF is identified. Caution patient not to "overlap" bolus doses, i.e., administer a correction bolus no sooner than 3 h after a rapid-acting insulin meal bolus and no sooner than 5 h after a short-acting insulin meal bolus. The 1800 or 1500 Rule may be applicable and may need to be recalculated if the patient's pump TDD has changed. (For ISF calculations, see Chapter 4.)

References

1. Pickup J, Keen H: Continuous subcutaneous insulin infusion at 25 years: evidence base for the expanding use of insulin pump therapy in type 1 diabetes. *Diabetes Care* 25:593–98, 2002
2. Lenhard MJ, Reeves GD: Continuous subcutaneous insulin infusion: a comprehensive review of insulin pump therapy. *Archives of Internal Medicine* 161:2293–300, 2001
3. Bode BW, Sabbah HT, Gross TM, Fredrickson LP, Davidson PC: Diabetes management in the new millennium using insulin pump therapy. *Diabetes/Metabolism Research and Reviews* 18 (Suppl. 1):514–20, 2002
4. Gabbe SG: New concepts and applications in the use of the insulin pump during pregnancy. *Journal of Maternal-Fetal Medicine* 9:42–45, 2000
5. Bending J, Pickup JC: Complications of insulin infusion pump therapy (Letter). *JAMA* 253:2644–2645, 1985
6. Walsh J, Roberts R: *Pumping Insulin*. 3rd ed. San Diego, CA, Torrey Pines Press, 2000
7. American Diabetes Association: National Standards for Diabetes Self-Management Education (Standards and Review Criteria). *Diabetes Care* 25 (Suppl. 1):S140–47, 2002
8. Farkas-Hirsch R: Insulin infusion pump therapy: keys to patient support in office practice. *Practical Diabetol* 11:24–27, 1992

9. Kaufman F, Halverson MJ, Lohry J: *Putting Your Diabetes on the Pump*. Alexandria, VA, American Diabetes Association, 2001
10. American Diabetes Association: Postprandial blood glucose. *Diabetes Care* 24:775–778, 2001
11. Warshaw H, Bolderman KM: *Practical Carbohydrate Counting: A How-to-Teach Guide for Health Professionals*. Alexandria, VA, American Diabetes Association, 2001
12. Davidson PC: Bolus and supplemental insulin. In *The Insulin Pump Therapy Book: Insights From the Experts*. Fredrickson L, Ed. Sylmar, CA, Mini-Med Technologies, 1995, p. 64
13. Bode BW, Steed RD, Davidson PC: Reduction in severe hypoglycemia with long-term continuous subcutaneous insulin infusion. *Diabetes Care* 19:324–27, 1996
14. Boland EA, Grey M, Oesterle A, Fredrickson L, Tamborlane WV: Continuous subcutaneous insulin infusion: a new way to lower risk of severe hypoglycemia, improve metabolic control, and enhance coping in adolescents with type 1 diabetes. *Diabetes Care* 22:1779–1784, 1999
15. Hirsch IB, Farkas-Hirsch R, Cryer PD: Continuous subcutaneous insulin infusion for the treatment of diabetic patients with hypoglycemia unawareness. *Diabetes, Nutrition & Metabolism* 4:41–43, 1991
16. Fanelli CG, Epifano L, Rambotti AM, Pampanelli S, Di Vincenzo A, Modarelli E, Lepore M, Annibale B, Ciofetta M, Bottini P, Porcellati F, Scionti L, Santeusanio F, Brunetti P, Bolli GB: Meticulous prevention of hypoglycemia normalizes the glycemic thresholds and magnitude of most of neuroendocrine responses to, symptoms of, and cognitive function during hypoglycemia in intensively treated patients with short-term IDDM. *Diabetes* 42:1683–1688, 1993

Resources

PUMP MANUFACTURERS

Pump manufacturers provide specific guidelines for pump therapy initiation as well as the use of their pump(s). All manufacturers distribute pump supplies and accessories. Some manufacturers provide distribution and service to Europe and Asia.

Animas Corporation
590 Lancaster Avenue
Frazer, PA 19355
1-877-YES-PUMP (1-877-937-7867)
610-644-8990
www.animascorp.com

Disetronic Medical Systems, Inc.
5151 Program Avenue
St. Paul, MN 55112
1-800-280-7801
763-795-5200
www.disetronic-usa.com

Medtronic MiniMed
18000 Devonshire Street
Northridge, CA 91325
1-800-MINIMED (1-800-646-4633)
818-362-5958
www.minimed.com

Sooil Development Company, Ltd.
196-1 Dogok-Dong
Kangnam-Gu
Seoul, Korea
82-2-3463-0041
www.sooil.com
Distributed in the U.S. by:
DANA Diabecare USA
2601 N. Hullen Street
Suite 100
Metairie, LA 70002
1-866-342-2322
504-889-9656
www.danapumps.com

Pump Supplies

Hypoguard USA, Inc.
One Corporate Center IV
7301 Ohms Lane
Edina, MN 55439
1-800-818-8877
www.hypoguard.com

Pump Accessories

Unique Accessories, Inc.
1625 Larimer Street
Suite 1206
Denver, CO 80202
1-800-831-8929
303-607-1298
www.uniaccs.com

Sample Forms

All pump manufacturers provide brand-specific pump training checklists, troubleshooting guides, and log forms, as well as the items included here. The educator or Certified Pump Trainer will be happy to provide the original or a photocopy of the patient's training checklist for your patient record.

The following forms may adapted to suit your needs:

PHYSICIAN/CLINICIAN FORMS

File these forms in the patient's record.

Insulin Pump Therapy Initiation Checklist

- Used to record patient's readiness/preparation for pump therapy.
- Physician and/or CDE completes during pump education process.

Insulin Pump Therapy Physician Orders

- Used to record prepump insulin regimen changes and orders for pump start.

■ Physician completes and provides to CDE and/or Certified Pump Trainer at least 5 days before pump start.

Insulin Pump Therapy Telephone Follow-Up

■ Used to record telephone information from patient during pump initiation period.

■ Physician or CDE uses to record patient's SMBG results, carbohydrate intake, and bolus doses during pump initiation.

PATIENT FORMS

Provide to patient/parent of child patient.

Insulin Pump Therapy Preparation Guidelines

■ Used to provide insulin changes/regimen and overall guidelines before and during the day of pump start. Complete several days in advance of start date. Photocopy after completion and file in patient's record.

Insulin Pump Therapy Start Guidelines

■ This form summarizes the patient's pump start regimen and instructions.

■ Complete and provide on day of pump start. Photocopy after completion and file in patient's record.

Insulin Pump Therapy Record

■ This is a 1-day log form to record SMBG readings, carbohydrate intake, carbohydrate bolus doses, correction bolus doses, and any other pertinent information that may affect target goals.

■ You may want to make several photocopies to provide to patient.

■ Patient uses this form to telephone or fax information to the clinician.

INSULIN PUMP THERAPY INITIATION CHECKLIST

Name _____ Pump start/training date _____

Pump brand/model _____ Serial number(s) _____

Saline trial?   No _____   Yes _____   (dates) _____

Diabetes Knowledge/Skills Training

Understands/demonstrates: Clinician   Date

❑ Rationale of self-management using pump therapy   _____   _____

❑ Benefits and challenges of pump therapy   _____   _____

❑ Need for frequent SMBG   _____   _____

❑ Target glucose levels (has targets)   _____   _____

❑ Carbohydrate counting (has insulin-to-carbohydrate ratio[s])   _____   _____

❑ Ability to use sensitivity/correction factor (has factor)   _____   _____

❑ Ability to calculate meal/snack bolus doses   _____   _____

❑ Treatment of acute complications   _____   _____

❑ Willingness to comply with medical recommendations   _____   _____

❑ Psychosocial adjustment (realistic expectations)   _____   _____

❑ Financial resources for pump/supplies   _____   _____

❑ Ability to use resources, e.g., support group, Internet   _____   _____

Pump Therapy Training

In addition to completion of the pump training checklist with the Certified Pump Trainer, understands:

❑ Infusion site selection, preparation, and hygiene

❑ Infusion set insertion and removal   Set type(s) _____

❑ Issues of daily living, e.g., wearing the pump, showering/bathing

❑ Exercise management guidelines

❑ Sick day management guidelines

  ○ Ketone test strips (has unexpired strips)

❑ Supplies to carry

❑ Troubleshooting guidelines

  ○ Prevention and treatment of hypoglycemia

- ○ Need for glucagon prescription and/or unexpired glucagon
- ○ Use of glucagon by family member/significant other

  Name:_____
- ○ Prevention and treatment of hyperglycemia
- ○ Diabetic ketoacidosis
- ○ Time off the pump (has conventional therapy regimen)
- ○ Who to call for help (physician, educator [RN, RD, RPh, psychologist], pump manufacturer help line, pump manufacturer customer service)

❑ Pump therapy follow-up guidelines
- ○ Who to contact for follow-up during pump initiation period
- ○ What to record: SMBG results, carbohydrate intake, bolus doses, activity, etc.
- ○ When to contact follow-up staff: how often, times
- ○ How to contact follow-up staff (phone, fax, e-mail)
- ○ Next office appointment scheduled for _____

  with _____

❑ Attach copy of Certified Pump Trainer Training Checklist to maintain in patient record form.

INSULIN PUMP THERAPY PHYSICIAN ORDERS

_____, MD

Patient _____ **Date** _____

Pump start date _____ **Brand/model**_____

Saline start?   No _____   Yes _____

Provide prescription for saline to patient

Saline start date _____ continue to _____

Insulin for pump _____ Humalog _____ NovoLog _____ Regular_____ Velosulin BR

Insulin regimen before pump start
❑ **Rapid-/short-acting insulin with glargine**

 ○ Discontinue glargine _____ hours before pump start

 ○ Continue injections of rapid-/short-acting insulin every _____ hours before
   pump start

 ○ _____

❑ **Rapid-/short-acting insulin with ultralente**

 ○ Discontinue ultralente _____ hours before pump start

 ○ Continue injections of rapid-/short-acting insulin every _____ hours before
   pump start

 ○ _____

❑ **Rapid-/short-acting insulin with NPH or lente**

 ○ Discontinue NPH/lente _____ hours before pump start

 ○ Continue injections of rapid-/short-acting insulin every _____ hours before
   pump start

 ○ _____

❑ **If on pump therapy and switching to another brand/model of pump**

 ○ Continue current basal rates and bolus regimen

 ○ Other (as indicated below)

Day of pump start

❑ Take usual dose of rapid-/short-acting insulin without lente, NPH, ultralente, or glargine

❑ _____

Starting basal rate(s)

❑ _____ units/h (24 h

❑ Other:

    Rate 1: 12 a.m. to ____ a.m.: units/h

    Rate 2: _____ units/h

    Rate 3: _____ units/h

    Rate 4: _____ units/h

Target glucose levels

Nocturnal _____ a.m. _____ mg/dl

Fasting/premeal _____ mg/dl

_____ h postmeal _____ mg/dl

Bedtime _____ mg/dl

Insulin-to-carbohydrate ratio

Bolus 1 unit for _____ g carbohydrate

Insulin sensitivity/correction factor

Bolus 1 unit for every _____ mg/dl >target

Infusion set change

Change site and set every _____ to _____ days

_____, **MD**   **Phone** _____
prescribing physician

INSULIN PUMP THERAPY TELEPHONE CALL FOLLOW-UP

Patient _____ Date _____

_____ Called as requested   _____ Called because _____

_____ Was called by me

           _____ To return patient's call   _____ Because patient did not call as requested

Current pump therapy regimen

Pump:

_____ Animas _____ Disetronic _____ MiniMed _____ Sooil _____ Model: _____

Insulin: _____ Humalog _____ NovoLog _____ Regular _____ Velosulin BR

Basal rates:

(1) 12 a.m. to _____ a.m.: _____ units/h

(2) _____.m. to _____.m.: _____ units/h

(3) _____.m. to _____.m.: _____ units/h

(4) _____.m. to _____.m.: _____ units/h

(5) _____.m. to _____.m.: _____ units/h

Insulin:carbohydrate ratio   **Insulin sensitivity factor**

_____ 1 unit:15 g   Add 1 unit for _____ mg/dl > _____ mg/dl

_____ 1 unit:12 g   Subtract 1 unit for blood glucose < _____ mg/dl

_____ 1 unit:10 g

_____ 1 unit:_____ gm

SMBG record using _____ meter

Date	Time	Blood glucose (mg/dl)	Carbohydrate (g)	Bolus (units)	Comments

Assessment _____

_____

Plan

_____ Continue current regimen

_____ Change regimen to:

12 a.m. to _____.m.: _____ units/h

_____.m. to _____.m.: _____ units/h

_____.m. to _____.m.: _____ units/h

_____.m. to _____.m.: _____ units/h

_____.m. to _____.m.: _____ units/h

Insulin:carbohydrate ratio   Insulin sensitivity factor

_____ 1 unit:15 g   Add 1 unit for _____ mg/dl > _____ mg/dl

_____ 1 unit:12 g   Subtract 1 unit for blood glucose < _____ mg/dl

_____ 1 unit:10 g

_____ 1 unit:_____ gm

_____ Change SMBG regimen to _____

_____ Patient to call (date) _____ with SMBG results

_____ Patient scheduled with _____ on (date) _____

_____, MD/CDE

INSULIN PUMP THERAPY PREPARATION GUIDELINES

Name _____ Pump start date _____

Congratulations on your decision to start insulin pump therapy!

Before your pump start day
❑ Check all the contents of your pump box and make sure you have everything as indicated on the shipping list. Call the pump manufacturer with any problems.

❑ Review the user's manual and watch the instructional video.

❑ Confirm pump start date, time, and location with your educator or Certified Pump Trainer.

Certified Pump Trainer _____Phone_____

Time _____Location _____Phone _____

Insulin regimen
❑ _____hours before your pump start, discontinue

○ Lente or NPH injection(s)

○ Glargine or ultralente injection(s)

❑ Take _____ units of _____ _____hours before pump start

❑ Continue injections of your rapid-/short-acting insulin _____, including the morning of pump start day

❑ _____

❑ Use your insulin sensitivity/correction factor to correct a high glucose reading

○ 1 unit lowers my glucose _____ mg/dl

Glucose monitoring
❑ Continue to monitor your glucose as usual

❑ The night before your pump start day, add a middle-of-the-night glucose check at

_____ a.m. and correct if > _____ mg/dl

Pump start day: Allow 3 hours for training
❑ Monitor your glucose and eat your usual breakfast

❑ Inject your dose of rapid-/short-acting _____ insulin to cover your breakfast

○ Use your insulin-to-carbohydrate ratio of 1 unit for _____ g carbohydrate

○ Correct a high blood glucose level, as needed, with your insulin sensitivity factor

❑ Wear comfortable, two-piece clothing for your pump start

❏ Bring:

○ _____ insulin (new, full vial) as prescribed by your physician

○ Insulin pump with all supplies sent to you, including:
  • Pump user's manual and any literature, warranty information, etc.
  • Pump batteries
  • Pump cartridges/reservoirs
  • Skin prep products
  • Infusion sets and dressings/tapes

○ Glucose meter, strips/sensors, lancets and lancing device

○ Calculator

○ Pen and paper

○ Food (lunch or snack)

_____, **MD/CDE**

INSULIN PUMP THERAPY START GUIDELINES

Patient _____ **Date** _____

Congratulations on your decision to start insulin pump therapy!

The following guidelines will help you during this start-up period:

Check your blood glucose six to eight times daily. Keep a record of the glucose results, amount of carbohydrate consumed, and your bolus doses. Use any log book or form of your choice. Refrain from moderate to intensive exercise during this time. We will be speaking daily during the next few weeks, so please remember this when planning your schedule.

Insulin type: ___ Humalog ___ NovoLog ___ Regular ___ Velosulin BR

Basal rate: _____ units/hour. You will start with one rate for 24 h. This rate will be changed as needed.

Diet: Follow your usual diet, using **carbohydrate counting**. Use your **insulin-to-carbohydrate ratio** of 1 unit insulin for ___ grams of carbohydrate. During your pump initiation period, until otherwise advised, please **omit** alcohol; Chinese and Mexican food; high-fat foods, including pizza, doughnuts, pastries, snack "cakes," pie, cake, and chocolate candy; and foods not usually consumed.

Bolus: Cover the carbohydrate you consume using your insulin-to-carbohydrate ratio, as described above. *Example:* You plan to eat 45 g carbohydrate, and your ratio is 1 unit for every 15 g. You would need to take an insulin bolus of 3 units to cover the carbohydrate. Based on your blood glucose level at the time, you may need to make adjustments in your bolus doses using your insulin sensitivity/correction factor.

Target blood glucose (goal): _____ mg/dl

Insulin sensitivity/correction factor: For every _____ mg/dl over your target glucose, add 1 unit to your meal or snack bolus. *Example:* Your premeal target glucose is 100 mg/dl, and your correction factor is 50 mg/dl. Your premeal reading is 156 mg/dl. Because you are about 50 mg/dl over your target, you will need to add 1 unit to your meal bolus to help lower your glucose level of 156 mg/dl to your target of 100 mg/dl. For now, do **not** take a correction bolus between meals unless directed otherwise. For a glucose reading <80 mg/dl, subtract ___ unit(s) from your meal or snack bolus. Bolus for high glucose readings no less than 3 h from your last bolus unless directed otherwise.

Blood glucose monitoring: Please check and record your results at the following times:
3:00 a.m., fasting, before each meal or snack, 2 to 2½ h after each meal or snack, and bedtime.

Hypoglycemia treatment: Follow the **Rule of 15:** A quick-acting source of 15 g carbohydrate, such as three glucose tablets, ½ cup juice, 8 oz skim/low-fat milk, or 4 oz non-diet soda, will raise blood glucose about 50 mg/dl in about 15 min. Recheck your glucose level after 15 min, and if you are still low, repeat the 15 g carbohydrate treatment. Try not to overtreat because overtreatment can create a vicious cycle of low blood glucose, too high blood glucose, bolus, etc. *Example:* Your blood glucose is 60 mg/dl. Drinking ½ cup juice will raise it to about 110 mg/dl in about 15 min.

Ketones: Make sure you have unexpired ketone test strips at home. Check for ketones when you have two consecutive blood glucose readings >240 mg/dl.

Infusion sets: Change your set and site every 2–3 days, as we discussed.

Call, fax, or e-mail your blood glucose, carbohydrate intake, and insulin bolus information **daily**, including weekends, unless directed otherwise.

Good luck! Remember, the next few weeks may be challenging, but learning pump therapy becomes easier every day, and all your efforts and hard work will be well worth it!

_____, **MD/CDE**

Phone _____ Fax _____ E-mail _____

INSULIN PUMP THERAPY RECORD

Name _____ Date _____

Current pump therapy regimen   **Target blood glucose** _____ mg/dl
Basal rates: 12 a.m. to ____ a.m. ____units/h
        _____.m. to _____.m.: ___ units/h **Insulin-to-carbohydrate ratio**
        1 unit:____ g
        _____.m. to _____.m.: ___ units/h
        _____.m. to _____.m.: ___ units/h **Insulin sensitivity factor**
        _____.m. to _____.m.: ___ units/h Add 1 unit for _____ mg/dl
        > _____ mg/dl (target)
        _____.m. to _____.m.: ___ units/h Subtract ____ unit(s) for blood glucose
        <80 mg/dl

	Noc-turnal	Pre-break-fast	Post-break-fast	Pre-lunch	Post-lunch	Pre-dinner	Post-dinner	Bed-time
Time								
Glucose (mg/dl)								
Carbohydrate (g)								
Carbohydrate bolus ___ unit								
Correction bolus ___ unit								
Total bolus ___ unit								
Activity								
Comments								

Notes

_____

_____

_____

_____

_____

_____

_____

Pump Tips
for Patients

GENERAL

1. Learn the proper terms and names that are specific to pump therapy, such as basal, bolus, prime, suspend, and brand-specific words. For example, refer to the infusion set tubing as just that, and not "the line."

2. Upon receiving your pump, review the user's manual and view the instructional video *before* the pump training session. Jot down specific questions and notes to ask the pump trainer.

3. Do not be afraid of your pump. You have total control over it; it will only do what you program it to do. Remember this, and you will develop more confidence the longer you wear it. Respect your pump, treat it with care, and learn how to make it do what you want it to do. There are lots of resources to help you.

WEARING OPTIONS

1. There are many options available for wearing the pump, including cases, clips, and pump-specific accessories, such as belts with pump cases, and leg garments. Check with the pump manufacturer for catalogs and suggestions.

2. Women may find wearing the pump in their bra, either under the arm in the bra side panel or inside the cup, may be comfortable. Control top panties or pantyhose also "anchor" the pump in place. Under dresses, the pump can be worn vertically in the small of the back. It can also be worn on the inside of the thigh under long dresses. For sports, women can place or tape the pump to the front center of a sports bra.

3. Wearing the pump inside the sock (using long tubing) works well for both women and men.

4. If wearing the pump under clothing, placing the pump inside an infant sock prevents moisture buildup and adds to comfort. Infant socks are available in a variety of colors; look for thin, cotton socks without a crew top to eliminate bulkiness.

5. For sleeping, try placing the pump in a specific location in the bed, such as next to you at your hip, clipped to the sheet or blanket, or inside a pajama pocket. You might like wearing a leg or armband. If placed under the pillow, the motor noise can be enhanced and may be disturbing. Restless sleepers may prefer longer tubing.

6. When showering with a nondisconnect infusion set, follow the pump manufacturer's guidelines. Your pump may come with special devices for showering or bathing to maintain water tightness. You can then place your pump inside a small, resealable plastic bag, attach string at the top corners to hang it up or wear around your neck, and cut the lower corners of the bag to allow water to drain out. Other options include placing the pump inside a suction-cup soap dish or shower caddy.

BATTERIES

When changing batteries, always remove and discard the dead batteries **before** opening up a package of new batteries. Placing new batteries next to the old batteries can cause confusion, and the new batteries could end up being discarded by mistake.

CARTRIDGE/RESERVOIR

1. When opening a cartridge/reservoir package, maintain sterile handling procedures. Placing the contents of the package on a paper towel makes viewing the contents easier and prevents rolling of the cartridge/reservoir.

2. When filling the pump cartridge/reservoir, tap the side forcefully to move any air bubbles. Push up on the plunger and make sure you see the air travel through the hub of the needle and out at the tip into the insulin in the vial. It may be necessary to draw in additional insulin and tap again to push the air bubble(s) out. As the insulin in the vial is used, gently slide the pump cartridge/reservoir needle down and out of the vial to keep the needle tip inside the insulin in the vial.

3. Calculate the amount of insulin required to fill the cartridge/reservoir, and remember that a vial of insulin contains 1,000 units. You may prefer to fill three cartridges/reservoirs at once, and refrigerate the two backups. Refrigerate the cartridges/reservoirs horizontally to prevent leakage.

4. Heat and temperature extremes can make the insulin less potent, causing high blood glucose readings. Insulin degradation can occur from the use of a Jacuzzi, sauna, or electric blanket. Anticipate the use of any of these, and fill the pump cartridge/reservoir accordingly, i.e., with only a few days' usage, not a full cartridge.

5. Always insert a new cartridge/reservoir with room temperature insulin. This step will prevent air bubbles from forming in the tubing.

6. Discard the cartridge/reservoir needle in a sharps container or other approved refuse container. An empty plastic bleach or detergent bottle can be used. Secure the lid with masking tape and dispose in regular, not recyclable, trash.

PRIMING

1. After priming, check the tubing daily for air bubbles. To remove air bubbles, if using a disconnect infusion set, disconnect the set from the site, prime the air bubbles out in midair, and then reconnect.

2. One inch of tubing contains 0.6 units insulin. If using a nondisconnect infusion set and a large area of air bubbles is present, the amount of air (noninsulin) can be calculated, and a compensatory bolus can be delivered.

INFUSION SETS

1. There are many different infusion sets. Many sets are compatible with different brands of pumps. Try different sets to

see what you might prefer. You may occasionally want to use a different infusion set for a specific reason. For example, a woman wants to wear a clingy knit dress and does not want to have a "bump" (the plastic base of her disconnect set) showing on her abdomen, so she opts for a nonbase needle set instead of her usual disconnect set. Work with your pump educator, and ask your pump manufacturer to send you samples of the various sets.

2. Select tubing length that is longer than the distance from your abdomen to the floor, so that if the pump is dropped or falls off the waistband/belt, the infusion set will not come out. Restless sleepers may prefer longer tubing. Longer tubing may also be preferred for showering because the pump can be placed in a soap dish or shelf during the shower.

3. The infusion set tubing does not necessarily need to be changed with each site change. You can purchase infusion sets with extra needles without tubing to control costs. Always change **both** the set and tubing if you have a site infection. "If in doubt, take it out."

4. If you find the insertion painful, try numbing the skin with ice, a cold can of soda, a cold spoon, or an anesthetic cream, such as Emla or Ela-Max. Keep in mind when planning your site change that the cream must be applied about 30 min before insertion.

5. **Always** change your site during daytime hours, when you will be awake for at least 4 h after the set change. Therefore, if you have a site problem or set kink, you will not sleep through the nondelivery of insulin.

6. When inserting the needle, stand up to prevent your skin from "bunching up" as you apply the dressing. Parents may find it best to insert the infusion set in a child who is lying down.

7. For sweating at the site, use an antiperspirant at the site, allowing it to dry before attaching the infusion set dressing or tape.

8. To prevent needles/catheters from coming out, use an adhesive, such as IV Prep or Skin Prep. Spray adhesives include Bard Protective Spray, Skin Prep, or 3M No Sting Barrier Spray. For stronger adhesion, try Mastisol, Skin Bond, or NuHope Adhesive.

9. To assist with set adhesion, an infusion set can be sandwiched between two layers of dressing: apply a dressing to the site first, insert the needle/catheter through the dressing, and then apply the set dressing/tape to the site's first layer of dressing.
10. To secure the tubing to the site, make a "safety loop" before applying the infusion site dressing. The set will be less likely to come out if pressure is exerted on the tubing.
11. A waterproof bandage, HY tape, or Hypafix dressings can help keep infusion sets in place during exposure to water. A knee-sized waterproof adhesive bandage can also be used to cover the infusion site.
12. If you have difficulty removing the infusion set adhesive after changing your site, try a commercial adhesive remover product, such as Uni-Solve.
13. If using a Teflon cannula disconnect set, remember to bolus immediately after applying the site dressing to fill the cannula. Follow the manufacturer's instructions. If you do not bolus to fill the cannula, you will miss part of your hourly basal rate, leading to high blood glucose levels.
14. Keep track of your site changes, and follow your health care professional's guidelines, changing every 2–3 days. Use a calendar specifically for this, and you will never have problems remembering when it is time to change. Remember, leaving the set in too long can cause poor insulin absorption, redness or tenderness at the site, high blood glucose levels, and, ultimately, tissue scarring.

PUMP SETTINGS

1. When setting maximum delivery amounts, remember to add a buffer amount for any potential increases in insulin needs, such as temporary basal increases, illness, or priming for air bubbles.
2. If applicable, practice use of the audio bolus feature. Try using this feature while wearing the pump hidden discreetly under clothing.
3. If the pump is able to display its screen in a choice of time limits, choose the longer time initially. This choice uses more battery power but provides a longer screen display during the learning process. As you become more comfortable with using the pump, you can revert to the standard display time.

4. Learn about all the features of the pump, such as a temporary basal setting, but remember to stick with using the basic features initially. The "bells and whistles" are there and can be reviewed and implemented after becoming comfortable with the basic functions of the pump. This step can take several weeks or months. Pump therapy is a process.

5. Keep records of glucose readings, carbohydrate intake, bolus doses, exercise, stress, and other factors that can affect diabetes control. Look for glucose trends and patterns. Some pumps can be programmed with more than one set of 24-h basal rates. It may be necessary to initiate different 24-h basal rates for gym/exercise, high stress, or premenstrual days.

6. When making basal rate changes or obtaining new basal rates from your health care professional, remember that **the pump clock always starts at midnight** (12 a.m.). *Example:* You have a regimen of three basal rates: 3 a.m. to 8 a.m.: 1.0 units/h; 8 a.m. to 4 p.m.: 0.7 units/h; and 4 p.m. to 3 a.m.: 0.8 units/h. This is actually a regimen of four basal rates because the start time of your first rate is midnight (12 a.m.). So, your actual basal rate program for 24 h is as follows: 12 a.m. to 3 a.m.: 0.8 units/h; 3 a.m. to 8 a.m.: 1.0 units/h; 8 a.m. to 4 p.m.: 0.7 units/h; and 4 p.m. to 12 a.m.: 0.8 units/h. To prevent any confusion, remind your health care professional to write any basal rate changes in this way, with the first rate starting at midnight (12 a.m.).

7. After setting your basal rates, **always** review the settings. Check start times and basal rate amounts. Verify your pump's total with your hand-calculated total: add up your basal rates for each hour of the day. Your total should match your pump's total.

8. With your pump educator, practice causing a warning/alarm to sound so you can recognize it when one occurs. Learn how to take action to silence the alarm and fix the problem **before** you have a problem.

9. Obtain a duplicate copy of your user's manual to keep with you when you are away from home. At the very least, photocopy sections that you might want to refer to, including the warning/alarm section, especially if you need to learn alarm codes.

10. Know who to call for each type of problem. For a medical concern, call your health care professional. For a pump

problem, call the pump manufacturer. Their toll-free number is located on the back panel of the pump. Always carry emergency pump supplies, too. This includes a syringe and vial of rapid- or short-acting insulin or an insulin pen.

BOLUS DOSES

1. To prevent forgotten bolus doses, decide on a specific meal/snack bolus delivery time, such as 5 min before eating.
2. Learn how to cancel a bolus during delivery **before** you need to do this. Practice so that you will know what to do. Also learn how to check your pump's memory to see how much of the interrupted bolus you actually received.
3. If your pump is equipped with a delay bolus feature, such as a Square Wave (Medtronic MiniMed) or Extended (Animas) Bolus, work with your health care professional to learn how to best use this feature. Pumps that do not have a delayed bolus feature accomplish the same thing by using a temporary basal increase because a delayed bolus is delivered during a pump's basal rate delivery. "Spreading the bolus out" over several hours of time may be helpful for gastroparesis, high-fat meals/snacks (such as pizza), high-fiber foods, and during parties or holiday meals. It may take several months of trial-and-error practice to develop a regimen that is right for you. Keep good records.

EXERCISE/SPORTS

1. When engaging in active sports, do not disconnect the pump for more than 1–2 h without taking any insulin. Get specific guidelines from your health care professional for each type of sport or activity.
2. Various levels of a sport require different basal rates. The basal rate change is affected by the duration and intensity of the sport, your current glucose reading, the desired target glucose level, the time and amount of your last bolus, and the time, amount, and type of your most recent meal/snack. It will take several months of trial-and-error practice to determine what works best for you.
3. Check with your pump manufacturer for suggestions on wearing your pump during physical activity. There are many options; obtain accessory catalogs for ideas.

SUPPLIES TO CARRY

1. Follow your pump manufacturer's guidelines for carrying supplies. At minimum, every day, carry at least *one* of each item you need to keep your pump working. This includes a complete set of batteries, insulin cartridge/reservoir, skin prep pad, infusion set, dressing/tape, vial of insulin, and medical identification card with emergency names and phone numbers. Additional helpful items include small folding scissors to cut dressing/tape, two Band-Aids (for additional dressing adhesion), alcohol pads to cleanse skin or dropped items, and an insulin syringe or insulin pen with cartridge for use in case of pump theft or total pump failure. Practice appropriate insulin storage procedures. Check insulin and battery expiration dates frequently, and replace your skin prep and alcohol pads often, too, so you are not surprised to open one that has dried out.

2. Backup pump items can be kept in a cosmetic or pencil bag, small craft box, or clear plastic resealable baggie. Office workers can keep an additional supply in their locker or desk. A vehicle glove compartment or trunk is another place to store necessary items. Use caution when storing insulin/insulin pens, and follow the manufacturer's instructions.

3. Pump therapy does not guarantee perfect blood glucose control, so remember to include treatment for hypoglycemia in your emergency supplies. Suggestions include glucose tablets, glucose gel, small juice cans or boxes, cake icing in tubes, small bags or boxes of raisins, and individually wrapped jelly candies (containing 12–15 g carbohydrate per piece).

Case Studies/
Success Stories

ROBBIE: SUCCESSFUL PUMP THERAPY
INITIATION IN AN ACTIVE TEENAGER

History

15-year-old 10th grade student
Age at onset: type 1 diabetes at age 9
Height: 5′ 10½″
Weight: 146 lb
SMBG: three to four times per day: premeal and bedtime (hs)
Ranges: 80–280 mg/dl; erratic control, nonspecific daytime pattern; fasting blood glucose (FBG) tends to be lower than other readings, 80–160 mg/dl
A1C: 8.2%
Physical activity: Soccer team 4 days/week in fall; swim team 6 days/week in winter; track team 4 days/week in spring; bikes 4 days/week in summer
Other: Frequent hypoglycemia after physical activity. Admits to overtreatment with excess cola soda. Posthypoglycemia treatment SMBG results are >350 mg/dl. Consumes 2,800-calorie exchange diet. Admits to "not always following and lack of understanding." Enjoys fast foods. Likes to sleep late on weekends

and takes morning insulin 3 h later than on weekdays. On weekends, FBG is always elevated. Has supportive parents.

Current insulin regimen

Lispro sliding scale:
<100 mg/dl: 2 units
100–150 mg/dl: 4 units
151–200 mg/dl: 6 units
201–250 mg/dl: 8 units
251–300 mg/dl: 10 units
301–350 mg/dl: 13 units
a.m.: s/s lispro (usual dose 4 units), 12 units NPH
Predinner: s/s lispro (usual dose 8–10 units)
hs: 16 units NPH
TDD: average 41 units/day

Pump therapy introduction

Robbie is frustrated with his current control and restricted mealtime regimen; he wants more mealtime flexibility and less hypoglycemia. He has a classmate who wears a pump and likes it. Robbie has concerns about wearing a pump during sports, especially swimming. He asks his parents and physician about pump therapy.

Pump therapy preparation

Clinician. Robbie's physician met with Robbie and his parents and explained pump therapy, demonstrated various water-resistant pump models and infusion sets, and provided written literature and pump information videos. She assessed Robbie's expectations and self-care abilities, reviewed/provided target blood glucose levels, scheduled carbohydrate counting sessions with an RD/CDE, and coordinated communication with a local CDE for pump follow-up and management. She later provided a pump prescription to the pump company for insurance coverage.

RD/CDE. The RD/CDE taught carbohydrate counting to Robbie and his mother, determined an insulin-to-carbohydrate ratio of 1:12 using Robbie's food diary and determined Robbie's ISF using his glucose records and the 1800 Rule (43 mg/dl rounded to 50 mg/dl).

Patient. Robbie reviewed pump information and videos; attended one local pump support group meeting, where he met a 27-year-old successful pump wearer and swimmer; obtained additional information on pump choices via the Internet; met with two pump company sales representatives; and chose a pump. Robbie's mother worked with the insurance and pump companies to obtain coverage for the pump and pump supplies. Robbie learned carbohydrate counting and practiced successfully for 10 days before pump initiation. Robbie was able to successfully calculate premeal lispro doses for fast food meals of cheeseburgers and milkshakes. SMBG results improved.

Pump therapy initiation

- Insulin-to-carbohydrate ratio is 1:12
- ISF is 50 mg/dl
- Do not use ISF for 3:00 a.m. SMBG
- Premeal target glucose is 100 mg/dl
- No after-school sports for 7–10 days

Prepump plan. Robbie's physician determined that Robbie's insulin regimen for 24 h before the pump start should consist of continuing the lispro dose and omitting NPH on the morning of the pump start.

Day 1

- Lispro insulin
- Basal rate: 0.7 units/h (24 h)

Clinician. Robbie's physician calculated the starting basal rate of 0.7 units/h × 24 h (41 units × 40% = 16.4 units ÷ 24 h = 0.68, use 0.7 units/h). She reviewed SMBG results, insulin-to-carbohydrate ratio, and ISF; provided rate and insulin information to the pump trainer and CDE; and gave Robbie and his parents pump initiation guidelines, including the need to omit after-school sports for 7–10 days during the basal rate adjustment period.

Patient. Robbie viewed the pump instructional video the evening before the pump initiation.

- 7:00 a.m. FBG: 202 mg/dl
- Took 6 units lispro to cover breakfast using 1:12 insulin-to-carbohydrate ratio; omitted NPH
- Completed a 3-h training with a pump manufacturer's pump trainer in his physician's office. Robbie's mother observed the training session and took notes.
- Pump therapy initiated at 12:00 p.m. with basal rate of 0.7 units/h

- 12:00 p.m. prelunch: 134 mg/dl; 53 g carbohydrate, 4.3-unit bolus, 0.7-unit correction bolus
- 5:45 p.m. predinner: 122 mg/dl; 67 g carbohydrate, 5.6-unit bolus, 0.4-unit correction bolus
- 10:00 p.m. hs: 143 mg/dl

Pump therapy follow-up and management

Robbie's physician used the services of a local CDE experienced with pump therapy to follow Robbie and make basal and bolus adjustments. Robbie called the CDE daily to report SMBG results, carbohydrate intake, and bolus doses. Robbie was reluctant to perform a 3:00 a.m. SMBG, but did so with his mother's assistance.

Day 2
- 3:00 a.m.: 132 mg/dl
- 7:00 a.m. FBG: 192 mg/dl; 42 g carbohydrate, 3.5-unit bolus, 1.8-unit correction bolus
- 11:30 a.m. prelunch: 111 mg/dl; 86 g carbohydrate, 1.2-unit bolus
- 6:00 p.m. predinner: 134 mg/dl; 55 g carbohydrate, 4-unit bolus, 0.7-unit correction bolus (underbolused for carbohydrate)
- 10:30 p.m. hs: 144 mg/dl

Day 3
Implemented second basal rate (would see results on Day 4):
- 3:00 a.m.: 139 mg/dl
- 6:45 a.m. FBG: 213 mg/dl; 42 g carbohydrate, 3.5-unit bolus, 2.2-unit correction bolus
- 11:30 a.m. prelunch: 156 mg/dl; 60 g carbohydrate, 5.0-unit bolus, 1.0-unit correction bolus
- 5:45 p.m. predinner: 128 mg/dl; 76 g carbohydrate, 6.3-unit bolus, 0.5-unit correction bolus
- 10:00 p.m. hs: 119 mg/dl
- Based on results 48 h after start-up, the CDE added a higher basal rate of 0.8 units/h from 3:00 a.m. to 8:00 a.m. to reduce dawn phenomenon blood glucose excursions.
- 12:00 a.m. to 3:00 a.m.: 0.7 units/h
- 3:00 a.m. to 8:00 a.m.: 0.8 units/h
- 8:00 a.m. to 12:00 a.m.: 0.7 units/h

Day 4
- 3:00 a.m.: 112 mg/dl

- 7:00 a.m. FBG: 154 mg/dl; 45 g carbohydrate, 3.8-unit bolus, 1-unit correction bolus
- 11:30 a.m. prelunch: 117 mg/dl; 75 g carbohydrate, 6.3 unit bolus
- 5:30 p.m. predinner: 96 mg/dl; 65 g carbohydrate, 5.5-unit bolus
- 10:00 p.m. hs: 123 mg/dl
- On Day 4, the CDE increased the 3:00 a.m. basal rate to 0.9 units/h.

Days 5 and 6
New basal rates:
- 12:00 a.m. to 3:00 a.m.: 0.7 units/h
- 3:00 a.m. to 8:00 a.m.: 0.9 units/h
- 8:00 a.m. to 12:00 a.m.: 0.7 units/h

An increase in the 3:00 a.m. to 8:00 a.m. basal rate to 0.9 units/h resulted in FBG readings ±30 mg/dl within the target level of 100 mg/dl. Robbie increased the frequency of his SMBG checks and continued to speak with the CDE daily the next several days.

Day 7
Robbie met with the CDE for a review of his SMBG results and observation of a site change. Robbie, his parents, the CDE, and the physician were pleased with his SMBG results. Robbie was now ready to resume his after-school sports.

Day 10
Sport days basal rates:
- 12:00 a.m. to 3:00 a.m.: 0.7 units/h
- 3:00 a.m. to 8:00 a.m.: 0.9 units/h
- 8:00 a.m. to 3:00 p.m.: 0.7 units/h
- 3:00 p.m. to 6:00 p.m.: temporary 50% decrease to 0.35 units/h
- 6:00 p.m. to 12:00 a.m.: resume 0.7 units/h

Ten days after pump initiation, Robbie resumed his after-school swim team practice and was instructed by the CDE to implement a temporary 50% decrease in his basal rate from 3:00 to 6:00 p.m. SMBG results were within target, and Robbie did not experience post-swim hypoglycemia.

Long-term follow-up
- Quarterly appointments with physician

▨ Annual appointments with RD/CDE
▨ Basal program
   12:00 a.m. to 3:00 a.m.: 0.7 units/h
   3:00 a.m. to 8:00 a.m.: 0.9 units/h
   8:00 a.m. to 12:00 a.m.: 0.7 units/h
▨ Basal total: 17.8 units
▨ Average TDD: 39 units

Robbie became accustomed to wearing his pump during swim practice but disliked wearing it for swim meets. He called the CDE and,
2 months after pump start-up, was advised to try disconnecting the
pump during the hour-long swim practice and also discontinue the
temporary 50% basal decrease. This proved to be successful. Robbie
continued to achieve SMBG results within his target range, with less
frequent hypoglycemia and hyperglycemia. He continued to sleep late
on weekends, and his weekend FBG results were similar to weekday
FBG readings, within target range. Three months after pump start-up,
Robbie's A1C dropped from 8.2% to 7.1%.

DEBORAH: SUCCESSFUL PUMP THERAPY INITIATION IN A FEMALE ADULT

History

38-year-old office manager
Age at onset: type 1 diabetes at age 26
Height: 5′ 3″
Weight: 136 lb
SMBG: usually 5–7 times/day: FBG, premeal, 2-h postmeal, hs. No
    specific pattern; frequent hypoglycemia
Ranges: FBG >200 mg/dl; premeal 50–270 mg/dl; postmeal
    150–320 mg/dl
A1C: 7.9%
Physical activity: Moderate exercises 2 days/week; 30-min walks
Other: Has mild retinopathy. States, "I'm either running high or
    low. I hardly ever have a normal blood sugar level, and I try
    really hard to do what's right." Was given 1,500-calorie diet
    7 years ago. Admits to, "I don't really follow anything specific. I
    thought I knew how to eat, but I think I need help. I'm tired of
    getting low blood sugars almost every day, and I have to eat
    when I don't want to." Husband is aware of Deborah's desire for

pump but questions her concern about wearing the pump and her ability to learn how to use it.

Current insulin regimen

a.m.: 7 units regular
Predinner: 5 units regular
hs: 32 units ultralente
TDD: 44 units/day

Pump therapy introduction

Deborah attended a local American Diabetes Association conference and visited the exhibit area. She saw insulin pumps at the booths and spoke with several pump manufacturer sales representatives and pump patients. Deborah read the information, watched the videos, and called her physician for an appointment. She had questions about wearing the pump discreetly under her clothing but liked the idea of eating when she desired instead of at specific times.

Pump therapy preparation

Clinician. Deborah's physician explained pump therapy in more detail. He suggested that Deborah meet with pump sales representatives and consider a saline trial because of her concern about "how to wear the pump." He referred Deborah to a RD/CDE to learn carbohydrate counting, provided a pump prescription to the pump company for insurance coverage and a saline trial prescription to Deborah and her pump trainer, and discussed switching Deborah to aspart insulin for pump therapy.

RD/CDE. The RD/CDE instructed Deborah in carbohydrate counting. She determined an insulin-to-carbohydrate ratio of 1:10 using the Rule of 450 and an ISF of 35 mg/dl using the 1500 Rule because Deborah was still using regular insulin and had not yet switched to aspart. The RD/CDE advised Deborah that she might need to do bolus checks after beginning pump therapy to determine whether the insulin-to-carbohydrate ratio needs to be changed with aspart insulin. She also arranged a follow-up appointment.

Patient. Deborah met with pump sales representatives and chose a pump. She worked with the RD/CDE on two occasions, learned and practiced carbohydrate counting for 1 month, and calculated breakfast and dinner insulin doses. Deborah realized she had not known which foods affected her blood glucose levels and had some improvements in glucose readings: all were lower, but the pattern was erratic. Her husband wanted to meet with the pump sales representative; therefore, an additional appointment was arranged. The appointment for pump initiation was arranged after the insurance company approved the pump. Deborah opted for a saline trial with her insulin pump. The week preceding her pump start with insulin she watched the pump instructional video and was trained by the pump manufacturer's pump trainer on the basic functions of the pump using saline. Deborah used her pump with saline for 3 days and wore it discreetly in the side panel of her bra. She delivered premeal saline bolus doses using the audio button feature of her pump while continuing her regular and ultralente insulin injections. Deborah thought the saline trial helped prepare her for "the real thing."

Pump trainer. The pump trainer instructed Deborah in basic pump functions and infusion site insertion using saline. She also provided tips on wearing the pump discreetly under clothing.

Pump therapy initiation

- Insulin-to-carbohydrate ratio 1:10
- ISF is 35 mg/dl
- Premeal target glucose is 120 mg/dl

Prepump plan. Deborah's physician determined an insulin regimen for the 36 h before the pump start. Deborah was instructed to continue prebreakfast and predinner regular insulin doses, discontinue ultralente 2 days before the pump start day, and add an a.m. dose of 15 units NPH and 12 units hs NPH.

Day 1
- Aspart insulin
- Basal rate: 0.75 units/h × 24 h
- Omit NPH dose and cover breakfast with regular insulin

Clinician. Deborah's physician calculated the starting basal rate of 0.75 units/h × 24 h using aspart insulin (44 units × 40% = 17.6 units ÷ 24 h = 0.73; use 0.75 units/h). He reviewed SMBG results, insulin-to-carbohydrate ratio, and ISF; provided rate and insulin information to the pump trainer; and gave Deborah pump initiation guidelines, including his fax number for follow-up. Deborah was advised to not use her ISF the first 2 days of pump therapy.

Patient. Deborah injected 6 units regular to cover breakfast and omitted NPH; she completed a 2.5-h training with pump manufacturer trainer in physician's office.

- 6:00 a.m. FBG: 241 mg/dl
- Covered breakfast using 1:10 insulin-to-carbohydrate ratio with regular injection
- Pump therapy initiated at 11:00 a.m. with basal rate of 0.75 units/h
- 12:00 p.m. prelunch: 166 mg/dl; 45 g carbohydrate, 4.5-unit bolus, 1.5-unit correction bolus
- 6:00 p.m. predinner: 88 mg/dl; 50 g carbohydrate, 5-unit bolus
- 10:00 p.m. hs: 216 mg/dl (no correction bolus)

Pump therapy follow-up and management

Deborah faxed or called her SMBG results, carbohydrate intake, and bolus information to her physician daily. He called her back each day with suggestions.

Day 2

- 3:00 a.m.: 222 mg/dl; no correction bolus
- 6:00 a.m. FBG: 229 mg/dl; 30 g carbohydrate, 3-unit bolus, no correction bolus
- 12:00 p.m. prelunch: 248 mg/dl
- Deborah called her results to the physician who advised her to use her ISF to correct the 12:00 p.m. reading. Took 3.6-unit correction bolus to reach target of 120 mg/dl
- 6:00 p.m. predinner: 64 mg/dl; treated with 15 g carbohydrate; ate 60 g carbohydrate, 6-unit bolus
- 10:00 p.m. hs: 137 mg/dl

Day 3

- 3:00 a.m.: 139 mg/dl
- 6:00 a.m. FBG: 124 mg/dl
- 11:00 a.m. prelunch: 156 mg/dl; 45 g carbohydrate, 4.5-unit bolus
- Deborah faxed her results to her physician who told her to continue her current regimen. Her physician began to consider a midday basal check test to determine whether the basal rate is too high or whether Deborah is using too large a bolus to cover her noon meal.
- 6:00 p.m. predinner: 55 mg/dl; treated with 30 g carbohydrate; 54 g carbohydrate, 5.4-unit bolus

■ 10:00 p.m. hs: 119 mg/dl

Day 4

■ 3:00 a.m.: 112 mg/dl
■ 6:00 a.m. FBG: 120 mg/dl; 45 g carbohydrate, 4.5-unit bolus
■ 11:00 a.m. prelunch: 136 mg/dl
■ Deborah faxed her results to her physician who recommended that she perform a basal rate check to determine whether the 11:00 a.m. to 6:00 p.m. basal rate should be decreased. Deborah agreed to do the basal rate check, which required her to omit her lunch and perform SMBG every 2 h until 6:00 or 7:00 p.m.
■ 1:00 p.m.: 111 mg/dl
■ 3:00 p.m.: 82 mg/dl
■ 5:00 p.m.: 63 mg/dl. Deborah (over)treated with 35 g carbohydrate and ate an early dinner.
■ 8:00 p.m.: 145 mg/dl
■ 10:00 p.m. hs: 138 mg/dl

Day 5

■ 3:00 a.m.: 141 mg/dl
■ 6:00 a.m.: 126 mg/dl; 45 g carbohydrate, 4.5-unit bolus
■ 11:00 a.m. prelunch: 140 mg/dl; 60 g carbohydrate, 6-unit bolus
■ Deborah faxed her results to her physician who advised her to implement a lower basal rate of 0.6 units/h 11:00 a.m. to 6:00 p.m.
■ New basal rates:
■ 12:00 a.m. to 11:00 a.m.: 0.75 units/h
■ 11:00 a.m. to 6:00 p.m.: 0.6 units/h
■ 6:00 p.m. to 12:00 a.m.: 0.75 units/h

Days 6–8
SMBG results within target range

Long-term follow-up

■ Basal rates:
■ 12:00 a.m. to 11:00 a.m.: 0.75 units/h
■ 11:00 a.m. to 6:00 p.m.: 0.6 units/h
■ 6:00 p.m.–12:00 a.m.: 0.75 units/h
■ Basal total: 16.95 units
■ Average TDD: 36 units

■ Quarterly appointments with physician
■ Annual appointment with RD/CDE

Deborah enjoyed pump therapy and was thrilled with the consistency in her readings. She felt more energetic, and lost 3 lb, which she attributed to a decreased intake previously consumed for treatment of her recurrent prepump hypoglycemia. Four months after the pump initiation, Deborah's A1C dropped from 7.9% to 6.7%.

ANDREW: SUCCESSFUL PUMP INITIATION IN A MIDDLE-AGED PHARMACIST WITH VARIABLE WORK HOURS

History

53-year-old hospital pharmacist who works three variable daytime shifts
Age at onset: type 1 diabetes at age 19
Height: 5' 11"
Weight: 186 lb
SMBG: seven to eight times per day: premeal, hs, and between meals during work hours
Ranges: FBG: 90–110 mg/dl; premeal: 130–180 mg/dl; hs: 110–160 mg/dl
A1C: 6.8%
Physical activity: Moderate physical activity; 1-h workout in gym using treadmill and running track 3 days/week
Other: Treated for adhesive capsulitis at age 46. Is satisfied with his level of control but struggles to maintain target glucose levels. Has been counting carbohydrate for past 2 years. Is tired of multiple daily injections and finds it difficult to adhere to insulin regimen because of variable shift work. Wants insulin pump for flexibility in lifestyle.

Current insulin regimen

Aspart insulin three times per day: prebreakfast, prelunch, and predinner
Insulin-to-carbohydrate ratio 1:5
Usual doses range: 10–15 units/meal
hs: 28 units glargine
TDD: average 64 units/day

Pump therapy introduction

Andrew knows several people using insulin pumps. His physician has also recommended pump therapy. Andrew learned about the various pump models by speaking with pump users, researching the pumps on the Internet, and comparing features in pump manufacturer literature and videos. He met with each manufacturer's sales representative and chose a brand. Andrew arranged to meet with his physician to discuss pump therapy initiation.

Pump therapy preparation

Clinician. Andrew's physician provided the necessary letter of medical necessity and prescription for insurance coverage.

Patient. Because he was already counting carbohydrate successfully, Andrew and his physician decided it was not necessary to meet with a dietitian. Upon receiving his pump, Andrew reviewed the user's manual and watched the instructional video. The pump manufacturer's pump trainer coordinated training in the physician's office.

Pump therapy initiation

- Insulin-to-carbohydrate ratio 1:5
- ISF is 30 mg/dl
- Premeal target glucose is 100 mg/dl

Prepump plan. Andrew's current MDI regimen simulated pump therapy. Because the hs dose of glargine acts as basal insulin, the bedtime glargine dose was reduced by 50% the evening before his pump initiation. Andrew injected 14 units glargine at 10:30 p.m. and was instructed to carefully monitor his glucose levels during the night.

Day 1
- Basal rate: 0.6 units/h until bedtime; increase to 1.2 units/h at bedtime (11:00 p.m.)
- Omit exercise at gym for 1 week.

Clinician. Because Andrew's usual glargine dose maintained his glucose levels within target, his physician calculated a starting basal rate of 1.2 units/h using the glargine dose as the basal rate (28 unit ÷ 24 h = 1.16, round to 1.2 units/h). Knowing that some of the preceding evening glargine dose may still be working during the first day of pump therapy, the physician initiated only 50% of the 1.2 units/h starting basal rate. Andrew's initial basal rate was calculated as 0.6 units/h, to be increased to 1.2 units/h at his bedtime, which was

11:00 p.m. The clinician instructed Andrew to call him each evening with his blood glucose and bolus dosages. He was told to continue using his ISF because it had proved successful with Andrew's pre-pump MDI regimen.

Patient

- 3:00 a.m.: 125 mg/dl
- 6:30 a.m. FBG: 116 mg/dl (within target range)
- Andrew used his insulin-to-carbohydrate ratio of 1:5 to cover breakfast. Andrew was trained by the pump manufacturer's trainer and completed the 3-h training by noon.
- 12:00 p.m.: 147 mg/dl; 45 g carbohydrate, 9-unit bolus, 1.5-unit correction bolus
- 6:00 p.m.: 156 mg/dl; 75 g carbohydrate, 15-unit bolus, 2-unit correction bolus (1.8 units rounded to 2.0 because of the pump's 0.5-unit incremental bolus function)
- Andrew called his physician, who advised him to continue his current regimen and reminded him to change his basal rate from 0.6 to 1.2 units/h at 11:00 p.m. Andrew did this.

Pump therapy follow-up and management

Day 2

- Basal rate: 1.2 units/h
- 3:00 a.m.: 111 mg/dl
- 6:00 a.m.: 74 mg/dl; 60 g carbohydrate, 11-unit bolus. Andrew calculated a 12-unit bolus but reduced it to 11 units because his glucose was in a low-normal range.
- 11:00 a.m.: 98 mg/dl; 45-g carbohydrate snack, 9-unit bolus
- 3:00 p.m.: 72 mg/dl; Andrew felt mildly hypoglycemic and treated with 15 g carbohydrate
- 7:00 p.m. predinner: 68 mg/dl. Andrew treated with 15 g carbohydrate; consumed 60 g carbohydrate for dinner, and used a 10-unit bolus to cover carbohydrate. He had calculated a 12-unit bolus but decided to reduce the bolus, thinking his basal rate may be too high. He called his physician, who agreed. Andrew was instructed to reduce his basal rate to 1.0 units/h × 24 h.
- 11:00 p.m.: 114 mg/dl

Day 3

- Basal rate: 1.0 units/h × 24 h
- 3:00 a.m.: 101 mg/dl
- 7:00 a.m. FBG: 121 mg/dl. Andrew overslept and skipped breakfast.

- 9:00 a.m.: 92 mg/dl; 30 g carbohydrate, 4-unit bolus. Andrew realized he miscalculated his dose; he had given 2 units too little. He decided to wait until lunchtime to see whether his glucose would be higher than expected.
- 12:00 p.m.: 165 mg/dl; Andrew took a 2-unit bolus to correct the high reading; 62 g carbohydrate, 12.5-unit bolus
- 6:00 p.m.: 114 mg/dl; 56 g carbohydrate, 11-unit bolus. Andrew called his physician, who was pleased with Andrew's results and advised him to continue his current regimen.
- 10:00 p.m.: 131 mg/dl; 1-unit correction bolus

Day 4

- 3:00 a.m.: Andrew forgot to perform SMBG
- 6:30 a.m. FBG: 108 mg/dl; 46 g carbohydrate, 9-unit bolus
- 8:00 a.m.: 126 mg/dl
- 11:30 a.m.: 118 mg/dl; Andrew was too busy to eat lunch; omitted noon meal
- 3:00 p.m.: 95 mg/dl; 50 g carbohydrate, 10-unit bolus
- 8:00 p.m.: 64 mg/dl; Andrew had drank two light beers during happy hour after work and munched on "a handful of pretzels." He did not take a bolus for the pretzels because he knew the alcohol might lower his glucose. He treated with 15 g carbohydrate and called his physician. Andrew was advised to continue the current regimen and avoid alcohol the next few days during his pump initiation period.

Day 5

- 3:00 a.m.: 144 mg/dl; 1.5-unit correction bolus
- 6:45 a.m.: 181 mg/dl; 2.5-unit correction bolus; omitted breakfast
- 8:30 a.m.: 262 mg/dl; Andrew called his physician, who asked him if he had changed his infusion site the preceding day. Andrew had not. He changed his infusion set and delivered a 5.5-unit correction bolus; consumed 45 g carbohydrate, 9-unit bolus.
- 12:00 p.m.: 116 mg/dl; Andrew was pleased with his reading and realized he must change his site every 2–3 days to prevent poor insulin absorption; 64 g carbohydrate, 12.5-unit bolus.
- 6:30 p.m.: 121 mg/dl; 66 g carbohydrate, 13.5-unit bolus
- 11:00 p.m.: 109 mg/dl

Days 6–8

Andrew's glucose levels remained within target. He occasionally miscalculated his bolus doses and used his ISF between lunch and dinner to decrease glucose elevations. He was able to skip some meals and eat at irregular times without adverse effects on his glucose readings. He was anxious to resume his exercise regimen and received his physician's permission to return to the gym.

Day 9

- 1 h before exercise, at 5:00 a.m., Andrew implemented a 3-h, 30% temporary basal decrease for exercise
- 5:00 a.m.: 114 mg/dl; 30% temporary basal decrease. Basal rate 0.70 units/h × 3 h (30% reduction of 1.0 units/h = 0.7 units/h)
- 6:00 a.m. to 7:00 a.m.: 1 h exercise on running track and treadmill
- 8:00 a.m.: 89 mg/dl; resumed normal basal rate of 1.0 units/h; 45 g carbohydrate, 9-unit bolus
- 10:00 a.m.: 72 mg/dl; 15 g carbohydrate
- 12:00 p.m.: 101 mg/dl; 54 g carbohydrate, 10-unit bolus
- 6:00 p.m.: 131 mg/dl; 60 g carbohydrate, 10-unit bolus, 1-unit correction bolus
- 11:00 p.m.: 94 mg/dl

Days 10–14

Andrew experimented with a lower temporary basal rate on his gym days (3 days/week). He reduced his 1.0 units/h basal rate by 40% to 0.6 units/h, and this reduction worked better than a 30% reduction. He had fewer episodes of hypoglycemia, and his glucose levels stayed within target range.

Long-term follow-up

- Quarterly appointments with physician
- Gym days: 40% reduction in basal rate implemented 1 h before to 1 h after exercise (0.6 units/h × 3 h)
- Basal rate(s): 1 units/h
- Basal total: 24 units/day
- Average TDD: 54 units/day

Andrew was able to eat meals at times according to his work shift without having to worry about injected insulin peak times. He was able to prevent postexercise hypoglycemia using a temporary basal rate decrease. His 3-month postpump start-up A1C level was 6.5%. Andrew felt he was able to maintain his excellent control with less effort than when using MDI therapy.

About the American Diabetes Association

The American Diabetes Association is the nation's leading voluntary health organization supporting diabetes research, information, and advocacy. Its mission is to prevent and cure diabetes and to improve the lives of all people affected by diabetes. The American Diabetes Association is the leading publisher of comprehensive diabetes information. Its huge library of practical and authoritative books for people with diabetes covers every aspect of self-care—cooking and nutrition, fitness, weight control, medications, complications, emotional issues, and general self-care.

To order American Diabetes Association books: Call 1-800-232-6733. Or log on to http://store.diabetes.org

To join the American Diabetes Association: Call 1-800-806-7801. www.diabetes. org/membership

For more information about diabetes or ADA programs and services: Call 1-800-342-2383. E-mail: Customerservice@diabetes.org or log on to www.diabetes.org

To locate an ADA/NCQA Recognized Provider of quality diabetes care in your area: www.ncqa.org/dprp/

To find an ADA Recognized Education Program in your area: Call 1-888-232-0822. www.diabetes.org/recognition/education.asp

To join the fight to increase funding for diabetes research, end discrimination, and improve insurance coverage: Call 1-800-342-2383. www.diabetes.org/advocacy

To find out how you can get involved with the programs in your community: Call 1-800-342-2383. See below for program Web addresses.

- *American Diabetes Month:* Educational activities aimed at those diagnosed with diabetes—month of November. www.diabetes.org/ADM
- *American Diabetes Alert:* Annual public awareness campaign to find the undiagnosed—held the fourth Tuesday in March. www.diabetes.org/alert
- *The Diabetes Assistance & Resources Program (DAR):* diabetes awareness program targeted to the Latino community. www.diabetes.org/DAR
- *African American Program:* diabetes awareness program targeted to the African American community. www.diabetes.org/africanamerican
- *Awakening the Spirit: Pathways to Diabetes Prevention & Control:* diabetes awareness program targeted to the Native American community. www.diabetes.org/awakening

To find out about an important research project regarding type 2 diabetes: www.diabetes.org/ada/research.asp

To obtain information on making a planned gift or charitable bequest: Call 1-888-700-7029. www.diabetes.org/ada/plan.asp

To make a donation or memorial contribution: Call 1-800-342-2383. www.diabetes.org/ada/cont.asp